WALL PILATES
WORKOUTS FOR WOMEN

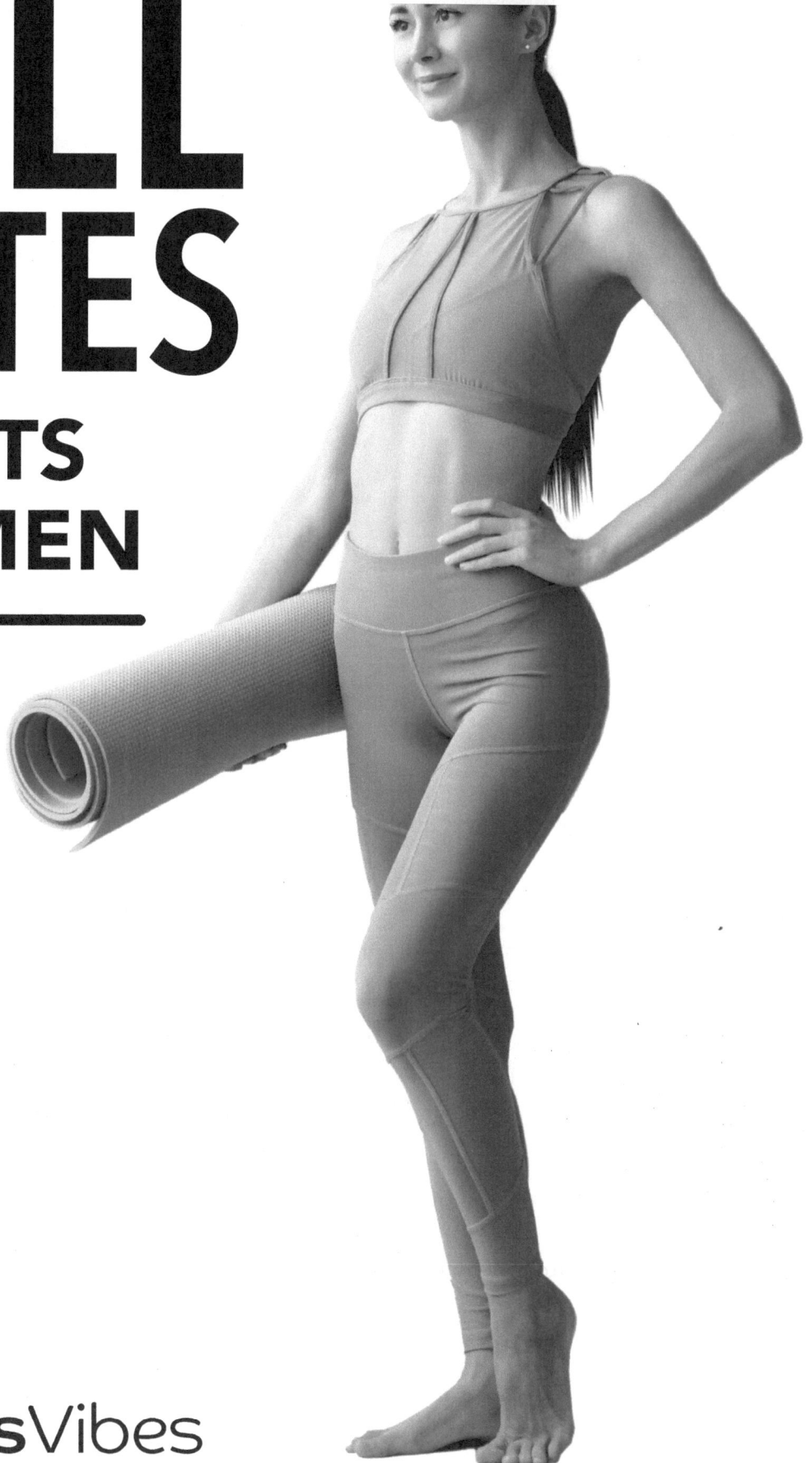

SheerFitnessVibes

TABLE OF CONTENTS

INTRODUCTION

Welcome to "Wall Pilates Workouts For Women"!

You've made a fantastic choice to enhance your fitness journey, and we're thrilled to guide you through every step. This book isn't just a collection of exercises; it's a pathway to improved well-being, strength, and flexibility, all centered around the innovative use of a wall.

We'll start with a quick introduction to Wall Pilates, which will guide you in setting up your space and preparing your mind and body for the workouts ahead, ensuring you get the most out of your practice!

After a brief introduction, we'll delve into the heart of the book where the excitement truly begins. The content explaining the practice is divided into three distinct sections:

- **Wall Pilates Exercises:** In this section, you'll delve into 45 Wall Pilates exercises, each meticulously detailed with accompanying tips and common mistakes to avoid. This guidance is designed to help you maximize the benefits from each movement.

- **Workouts and Routines:** This chapter transforms the exercises from the previous section into engaging 5-10 minute workout routines. Incorporate them into your daily schedule to establish a consistent habit. Feel free to tailor these routines by mixing exercises according to your preferences and fitness objectives!

- **28-Day Challenge:** Are you prepared for a transformative journey? Dive into this chapter's detailed 28-day workout plan, focused on boosting your energy and tonicity. Day by day, you'll engage in diverse routines, guaranteeing a varied and thorough exercise experience.

If you're still concerned about performing the exercises and workouts correctly, don't worry—we've got you covered! As promised, every exercise and workout in this book, including the 28-day challenge, is accompanied by a video tutorial to show you exactly how it's done. You can swiftly access this digital content by scanning the corresponding QR code, which will direct you to the specific exercise you wish to review. Alternatively, our comprehensive app is available for download on both Android and Apple app stores, providing easy access to all video tutorials.

Now, are you ready to feel leaner and stronger? Choose your wall, and let's begin!

ACCESS THE VIDEO TUTORIALS

In this book, alongside every exercise, you'll encounter distinctive small square patterns—these are QR codes. You might already be familiar with them, but if not, here are some quick instructions on how to use them.

Think of these QR codes as your digital gateways to insightful video content! A QR code functions similarly to a barcode. However, instead of being scanned at a checkout, you scan it with your smartphone or tablet, granting access to valuable visual guidance for each exercise.

Don't worry if you encounter any issues with the QR code or prefer an alternative method. You can always visit our website at **www.sheerfitnessvibes.com** to access the video tutorials. While our website features various sections, only the wall pilates section is available for _lifetime free access_ as a benefit of purchasing this book. This section is exclusive and requires a specific access code, which you, as a book owner, are entitled to receive. To activate your lifetime access to the wall pilates content, please turn to **page 112** and follow the provided instructions.

We've implemented these solutions to help you easily visualize and comprehend every exercise, whether you're using the QR code or visiting the website directly.

If you're new to QR codes, we encourage you to give them a try. They offer a straightforward way to enrich your learning experience and ensure you're performing each exercise correctly.

Now, are you ready to jump into this fitness journey? Let's get started!

1.

Open the camera on your smartphone and point it at the QR code for the exercise you wish to access.

2.

When you aim your camera at the QR code, a button should appear on your screen. If nothing happens, try tapping the area on your phone's screen displaying the QR code. Click the button when it appears.

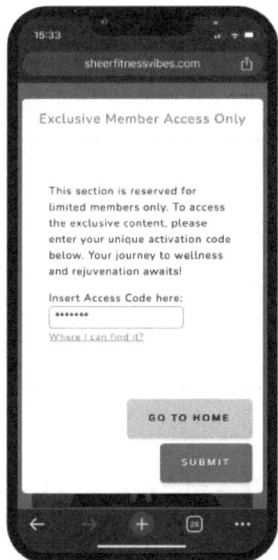

3.

You will be redirected to the video tutorial linked to the QR code. If you're using the device for the first time, you'll be asked to enter the code found on page 112. Don't fret; you'll only need to enter this code once for each device you use.

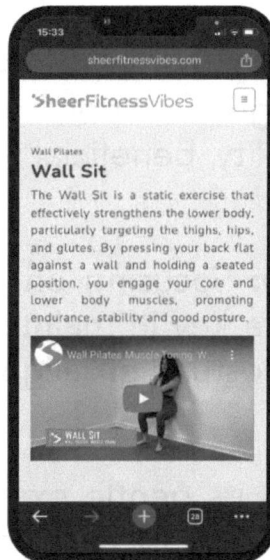

4.

Once you've entered the code, you'll have lifetime access to our video tutorials. If you encounter any issues, feel free to contact us at the following email address:

support@sheerfitnessvibes.com

MAKE THE MOST OUT OF WALL PILATES

WHY DO WALL PILATES?

Wall Pilates is a variation of traditional Pilates exercises that incorporates a wall as a crucial component to enhance the workout's effectiveness and provide additional support. It utilizes the resistance and support of the wall to deepen stretches, improve balance, and increase the intensity of various exercises. Why choose Wall Pilates over other workouts? Let's delve into Wall Pilates' key strengths:

- **Low-Impact Exercise:** Wall Pilates is renowned for its low-impact and gentle approach to fitness, offering safe workouts that are suitable for all ages and fitness levels.

- **Toning and Sculpting:** The exercises effectively tone and sculpt the body, targeting areas like the legs, glutes, arms, and abdomen while also focusing on belly fat reduction to help sculpt the silhouette you've always desired!

- **Core Strengthening:** Through Wall Pilates, you'll strengthen your deep core muscles, crucial for a stable spine and diminishing lower back pain, leading to better movement and stability in daily activities.

- **Enhanced Flexibility:** Using the wall as a prop can help deepen stretches and extend the range of motion beyond traditional floor exercises. This leads to improved flexibility, beneficial for overall movement efficiency and injury prevention.

- **Improved Posture:** Focusing on alignment and core strength, many Wall Pilates exercises are key in maintaining good posture. The wall's feedback aids in correcting postural misalignments, facilitating these improvements in daily life.

- **Accessibility:** With its gentle exercises and supportive feedback from the wall, Wall Pilates is accessible to individuals of any age, gender, and fitness level. Its blend of low-impact yet targeted workouts fit various body types and easily integrates into the busiest schedules, requiring just 10 minutes daily to start noticing benefits.

In conclusion, Wall Pilates stands as a beacon for individuals seeking a fitness regimen that is both nurturing and challenging, providing a versatile and adaptable approach to achieving personal health goals.

PRE-WORKOUT CHECKLIST

While Wall Pilates doesn't demand a lot of equipment, ensuring you have the right setup is key to a successful and safe practice. Set yourself up for success by ensuring these key components are at your disposal before starting:

- **Wall and Space:** The essential element for Wall Pilates is, of course, a wall. But it's just as vital to have enough surrounding space. Whether you're leaning against the wall or extending on the floor, ensure you have ample room to move freely. Clear any nearby clutter to establish a safe and calming environment for your practice.

- **Yoga Mat:** Essential for floor exercises, a high-quality yoga mat offers cushioning, traction, and delineates your workout zone. Choose one that provides enough padding for comfort and is grippy to prevent any slipping during your routines.

- **Light Dumbbells:** Incorporating a pair of light dumbbells can enhance your arm-sculpting exercises, adding an element of resistance to strengthen your muscles. While this book recommends using light weights for certain routines, you can easily substitute them with household items like water bottles or cans if dumbbells are not available.

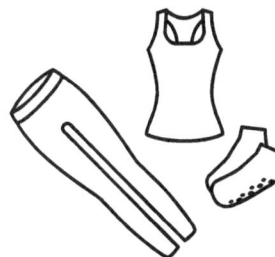

- **Comfortable Attire:** While not actual equipment, proper attire is essential. Opt for breathable, flexible, and snug clothing that ensures full movement and enables posture and alignment checks during exercises.

- **Anti-slip Socks (Optional):** Appropriate clothing can significantly impact your session. Opt for garments that are breathable, flexible, and snug, facilitating movement and allowing you to check your form and posture easily.

With this essential gear in hand, you're ready to unlock the full potential of Wall Pilates, setting the foundation for a transformative workout routine.

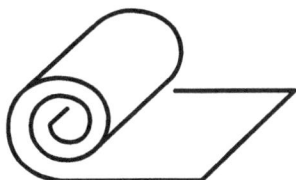

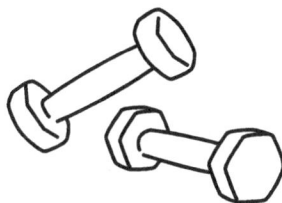

☐ **YOGA MAT**   ☐ **LIGHT DUMB-BELLS OR ALTERNATIVES**   ☐ **COMFORTABLE ATTIRE**

PREPARATION TIPS

While Wall Pilates is a low-intensity practice, some preparation is still essential.

Engage in Wall Pilates sessions on a relatively empty stomach, as a heavy meal can make you feel sluggish and may hinder your ability to perform deep abdominal contractions. If you need to eat, opt for a light snack about 30 minutes to an hour before your workout.

Staying hydrated is crucial, but avoid consuming large quantities of water immediately before starting your session. Excessive water intake can lead to discomfort and bloating during exercises. It's best to drink steadily throughout the day and have just a small amount of water 15-20 minutes before you begin. Also, avoid beverages that might impact your hydration status or energy levels, such as alcohol and caffeinated drinks, before your workout, as they can affect your balance, coordination, and focus.

Before you begin, dedicate a few moments to clear your mind and set your intentions for your practice. Mental preparation can significantly enhance your focus and the effectiveness of your workout. Use your Wall Pilates time to relax, release stress, and enjoy the process. A positive attitude can profoundly influence your results!

Lastly, it is **crucial to listen to your body**. Wall Pilates, being a low-impact practice, should not be overdone, or it may hamper your progress. The exercises in the upcoming chapter require proper form and alignment for effective execution. Overextending yourself could lead to poor posture and back arching, diminishing the exercises' benefits. Therefore, maintain focus, heed your body's signals, and respect your current limits. With regular practice, your capabilities will naturally expand.

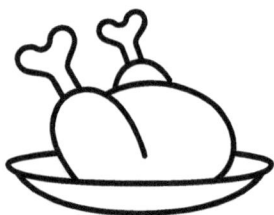

1 AVOID HEAVY MEALS PRE-WORKOUT

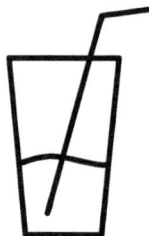

2 DON'T DRINK MUCH BEFORE SESSIONS

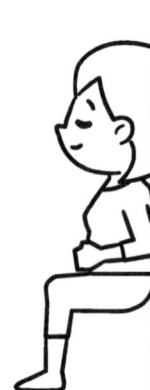

3 CLEAR YOUR MIND AND LISTEN TO YOUR BODY

THE COACH

Karen Martinez

Karen Martinez is a certified personal trainer based in London, known for her commitment to helping clients achieve their fitness goals through personalized and innovative workout programs. Karen offers a holistic approach to health and wellness, specializing in combining the latest fitness trends with traditional training techniques to ensure her clients not only see immediate results but also build sustainable habits for long-term health. Her passion for fitness and dedication to her clients' success make her a sought-after trainer for those looking to transform their lives through exercise and healthy living.

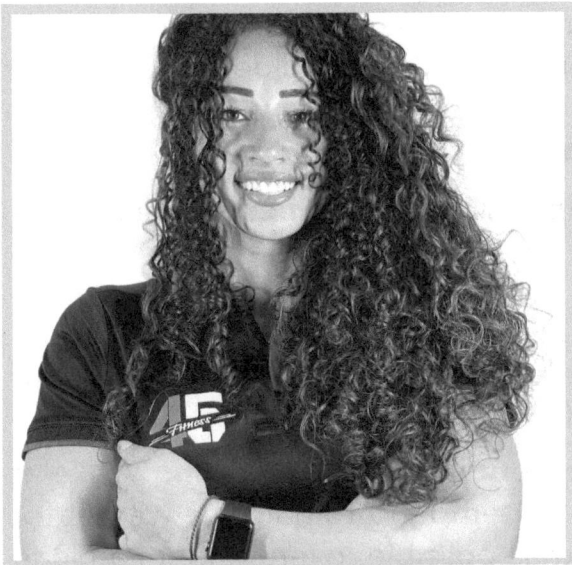

" *I'm dedicated to promoting health and fitness, always on the lookout for creative strategies to help my clients succeed. With a rich background in various training techniques and a strong educational foundation, I bring a comprehensive and innovative approach to each session. Let's embark on this journey together, transforming challenges into victories!* **"**

WALL SIT

INSTRUCTIONS

1. Begin by standing with your back against a flat wall, feet shoulder-width apart and about 2 feet away from the wall.

2. Slowly slide down the wall until your thighs are parallel to the ground, ensuring your knees are directly above your ankles and form a 90-degree angle.

3. Press your entire back flat against the wall, including the lower back and shoulders. Engage your core muscles to maintain stability.

4. Perform a slight chin tuck to align your head with your spine, looking straight ahead to maintain a neutral neck and spine position. Ensure your shoulders are aligned and relaxed.

5. Hold this position for 20 to 60 seconds, depending on your ability, while breathing deeply and steadily.

✓ **TIP:** Performing this exercise in front of a mirror can help you check the correct posture and alignment of your shoulders and legs.

✗ MISTAKES TO AVOID

- **Improper Knee Alignment:** Ensure your knees do not extend past your toes to avoid undue stress on the knee joints. Keep your weight evenly distributed between both feet and drive through your heels for added stability.

- **Overextending the Duration:** While it might be tempting to hold the wall sit for as long as possible, overdoing it can lead to muscle fatigue and poor form. Start with manageable durations and gradually increase as your strength and endurance improve.

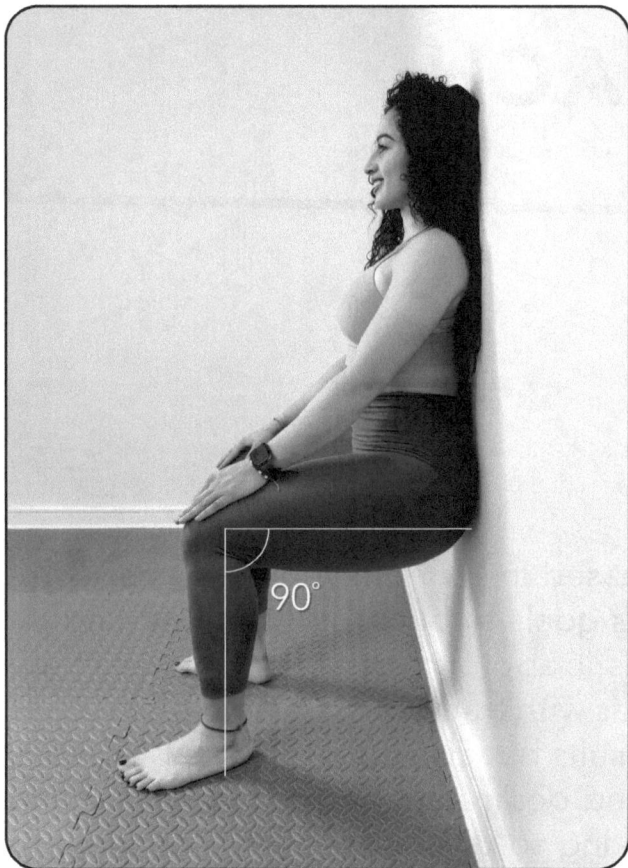

The Wall Sit is a static exercise that effectively strengthens the lower body, particularly targeting the thighs, hips, and glutes. By pressing your back flat against a wall and holding a seated position, you engage your core and lower body muscles, promoting endurance and stability. This exercise is also beneficial for improving posture; the alignment of the back and the slight tuck of the chin during the hold help reinforce a neutral spine position, contributing to better overall body alignment.

WALL SIT HEEL RAISE

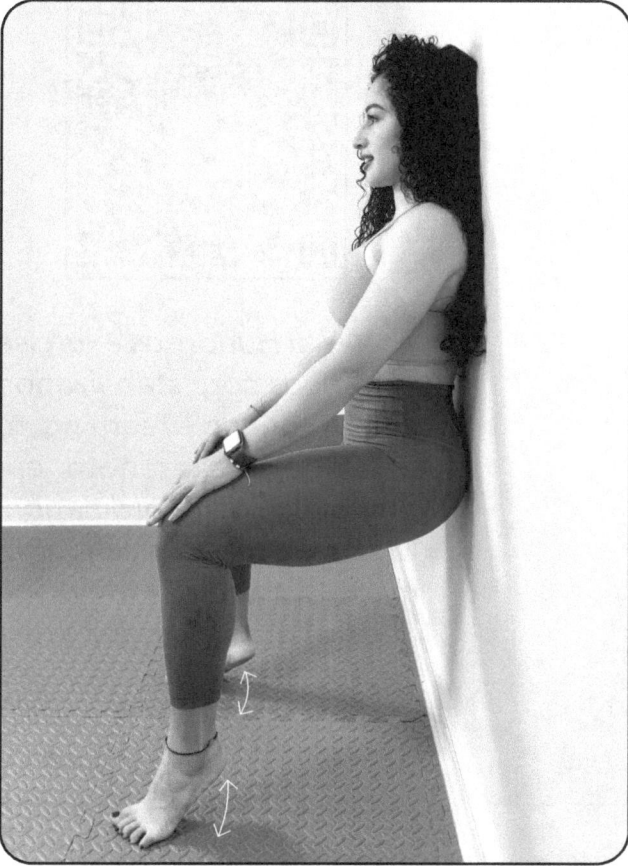

The Wall Sit Heel Raise is a variation of the traditional wall sit exercise, adding an extra movement that targets the calf muscles in addition to the quadriceps, hamstrings, and glutes. This variation not only strengthens the lower body but also improves balance and stability.

INSTRUCTIONS

1. Begin by performing the regular wall sit.

2. While maintaining the wall sit position, slowly lift your heels off the ground, rising onto the balls of your feet. Keep your core engaged and your back flat against the wall to maintain balance.

3. Hold the heel raise for a few seconds, then slowly lower your heels back to the floor.

4. Continue to lift and lower your heels for a set number of repetitions or for a certain duration, depending on your fitness level.

5. After completing the heel raises, slide back up the wall to return to a standing position and rest for a moment before repeating the exercise if desired.

✓ TIPS

- Focus on smooth and controlled movements.

- Keep your weight evenly distributed across both feet and ensure your knees remain aligned with your ankles, not extending past your toes.

✗ MISTAKES TO AVOID

- **Leaning Forward:** Avoid leaning your torso forward as you lift your heels. This can shift your weight improperly and reduce the effectiveness of the exercise. Aim to keep your back flat against the wall throughout the movement.

- **Rushing:** Take your time with each heel raise to ensure proper form and muscle engagement.

THE HUNDREDS

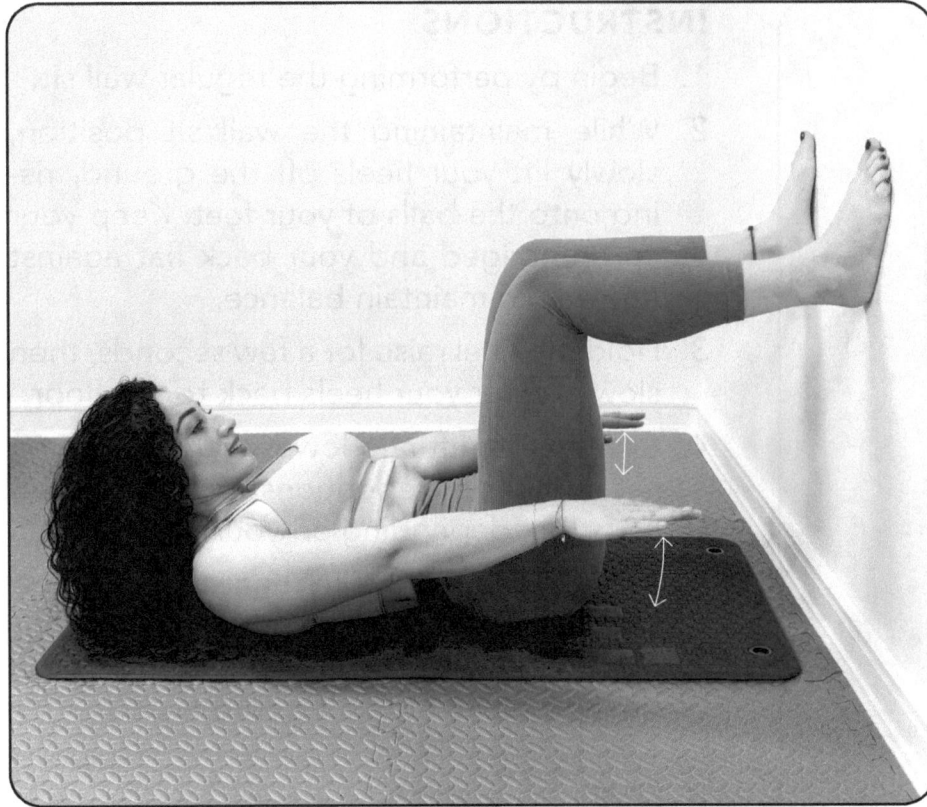

The Wall Hundreds exercise combines core stabilization with rhythmic breathing to enhance core strength, endurance, and coordination. Maintaining core engagement, spinal neutrality, and neck alignment during the 100 pulses is key for an effective abdominal and posture-enhancing workout.

INSTRUCTIONS

1. Begin by lying down on your back on a mat, facing the wall, with feet flat against the wall and knees bent at 90 degrees, ensuring your legs are hip-width apart. Maintain a neutral spine with your arms by your sides.

2. Inhale deeply, then exhale to engage your core, keeping a gentle curve in your lower back. Lift your head and shoulders, extending your arms towards your hips, palms down, and maintain a neutral neck by keeping your gaze towards your knees

3. Start pulsing your arms in small, controlled movements, coordinating your breath with the pulses: inhale for five pulses and exhale for five. Continue for a total of 100 pulses, keeping your core engaged.

4. Once you complete the 100 pulses, slowly lower your head and shoulders back to the mat and relax your arms by your sides.

✓ **TIP:** Ensure your feet remain firmly against the wall throughout the exercise to provide stability and support.

✗ MISTAKES TO AVOID

- **Losing Core Engagement:** Ensure your abdominal muscles are activated at all times to protect your spine and maximize the workout's effectiveness.

- **Incorrect Neck Position:** Keeping your neck improperly aligned can lead to neck strain. Maintain a neutral neck position by keeping your gaze directed towards your knees.

QUAD STRETCH

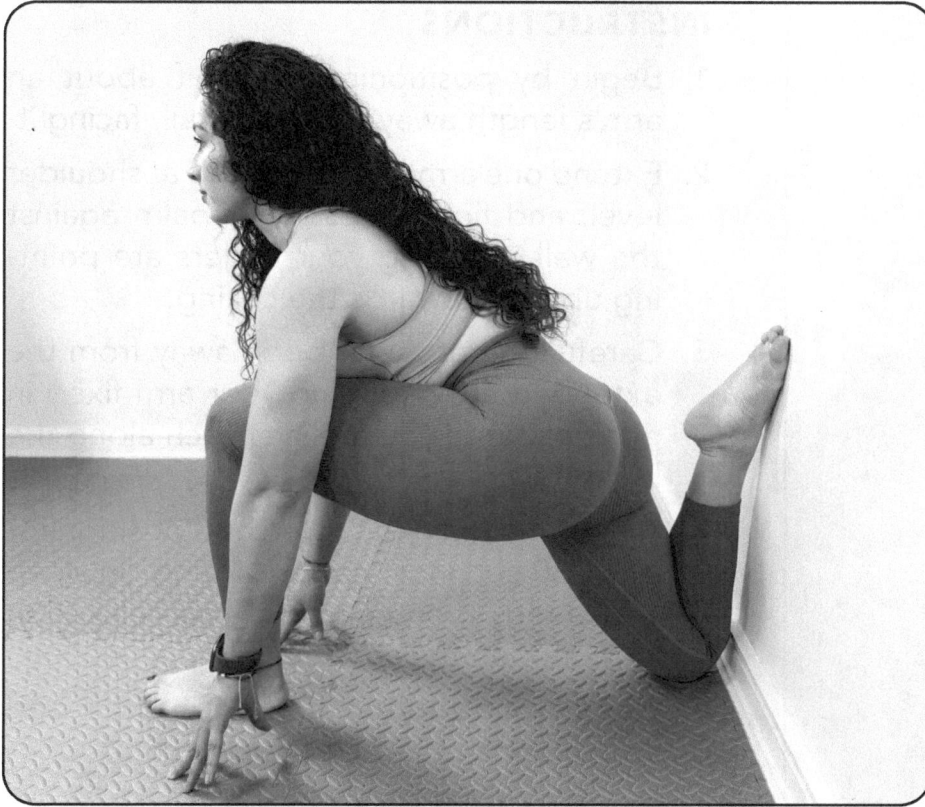

The Quad Stretch against the wall targets the quadriceps by having one leg bent against the wall behind you and the other foot flat on the floor in front, creating an effective stretch. This position helps improve leg flexibility, relieve muscle tightness, and support recovery.

INSTRUCTIONS

1. Begin by kneeling and facing away from the wall.

2. Move one knee back so that your foot's top, shin, and knee touch the wall. The closer your knee is to the wall, the more intense the stretch.

3. Step your other foot forward, placing it flat on the floor.

4. Gently lean forward, using your hands for support on the mat.

5. Hold the stretch for 30 seconds, breathing deeply. Focus on relaxing the quad of the back leg to deepen the stretch.

6. To release, shift your weight to your front leg and gently remove your back leg from the wall.

7. Switch legs and repeat the stretch.

✓ TIPS

- Place a towel or pillow under your knee against the wall for extra comfort.

- If you notice your back curving, straighten your torso and place your hands on your knee to achieve a more upright position.

✗ MISTAKES TO AVOID

- **Overextending the Front Knee:** Ensure the knee of your front leg doesn't pass your toes to avoid knee strain. Keep the knee directly over the ankle.

- **Forcing the Stretch:** Don't push into the stretch too hard. Aim for mild tension without pain. If you experience sharp pain, reduce intensity by stepping slightly away from the wall, which will decrease the stretch's depth.

BICEP STRETCH

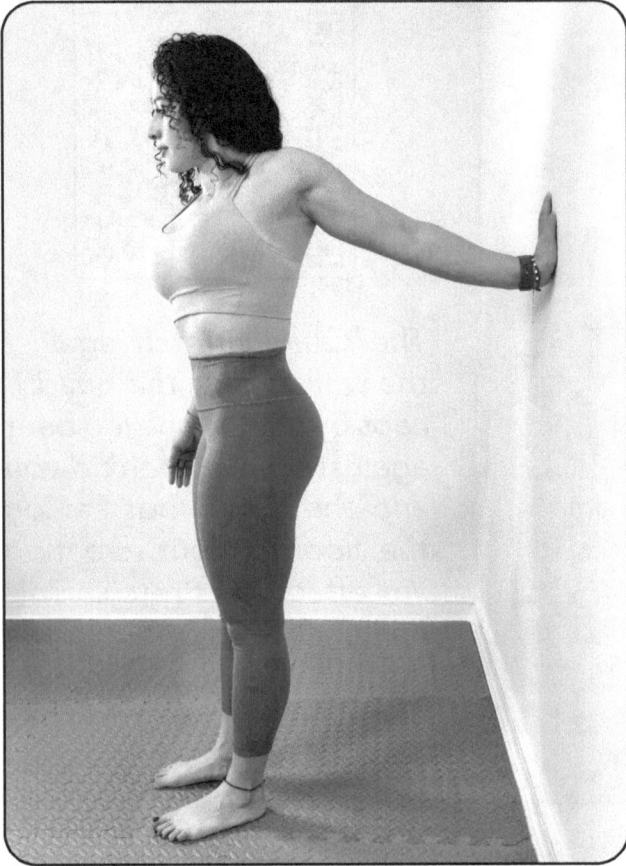

INSTRUCTIONS

1. Begin by positioning yourself about an arm's length away from the wall, facing it.

2. Extend one arm straight ahead at shoulder level, and firmly press your palm against the wall, ensuring your fingers are pointing upward towards the ceiling.

3. Carefully rotate your body away from the extended arm, keeping your arm fixed in position, until you feel a stretch along the bicep muscle.

4. Aim to maintain this stretched position for a full 30 seconds, concentrating on deep and steady breaths to facilitate relaxation and deepen the stretch.

5. Gently rotate to the starting position and switch arms to repeat the stretch.

✓ TIPS

- Start with a gentle stretch and gradually increase the intensity by rotating your body further, as long as there's no pain.

- Deep, steady breaths can help you relax into the stretch, allowing your bicep muscle to elongate more effectively.

✗ MISTAKES TO AVOID

- **Raising your Shoulder:** Keep the shoulder of the stretching arm down and relaxed. Raising the shoulder can create tension in the neck and shoulder area, detracting from the stretch's effectiveness.

- **Neglecting Posture:** Maintain a straight spine and avoid leaning towards the wall or twisting your body excessively, which can compromise the stretch and potentially cause discomfort or injury.

The Bicep Stretch against the wall is a simple yet effective exercise designed to increase flexibility and relieve tension in the biceps. It's an excellent way to counteract the tightness that can result from repetitive arm exercises, heavy lifting, or prolonged periods of desk work. Holding the stretch while focusing on deep, steady breathing helps to maximize the benefits, promoting relaxation and improving muscle elasticity. This stretch is ideal for inclusion in both warm-up routines and cool-down sequences, aiding in muscle recovery and injury prevention.

SIDE LEG RAISES

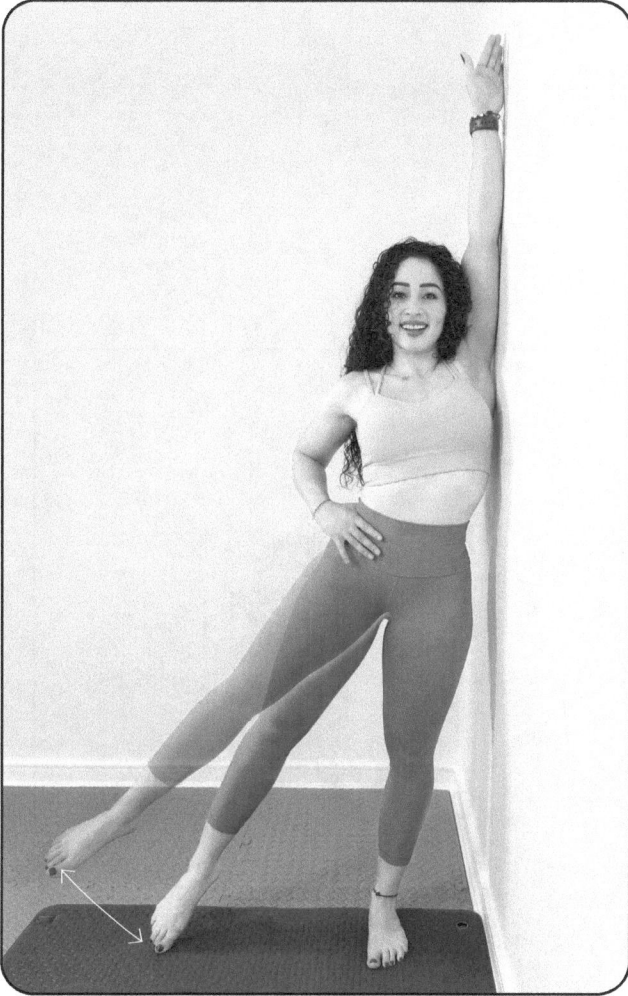

INSTRUCTIONS

1. Begin by standing parallel to the wall with your left side facing it. Raise your left arm above your head and press it against the wall for support, making sure your left side is also aligned and pressed against the wall.

2. Shift your weight onto your left leg, keeping it straight for stability.

3. Slowly lift your right leg to the side, maintaining a straight leg and ensuring your foot is flexed and pointing forward.

4. Raise your leg as high as comfortably possible without compromising your posture, then slowly lower it back down with control, lightly touching the floor with your toe before lifting again.

5. Repeat lifting your leg for 30 seconds, emphasizing smooth, controlled motions and deep breaths.

6. After finishing the set, switch sides by turning around so your right side is against the wall. Repeat the exercise with your left leg.

✓ TIPS

- Engage your core to maintain balance and enhance the stability of the movement.
- For an added challenge, pause at the top of the leg raise.

✗ MISTAKES TO AVOID

- **Bending Your Knees:** Keep the leg you're lifting straight. Bending your knee can reduce the effectiveness of the exercise.
- **Raising Your Leg Too High:** Focus on controlling the motion rather than achieving maximum height. Lifting your leg too high can compromise your posture and lead to loss of balance or strain.

The Side Leg Raises with an opposite side stretch against the wall not only effectively strengthen the hips, thighs, and glutes but also stretch the opposing side's muscles, offering a dual benefit. This dynamic movement enhances hip mobility and leg stability while also delivering a deep, beneficial stretch to the torso and side muscles. Additionally, by engaging both the lower and upper body, this exercise promotes overall balance and posture, making it an integral part of a holistic fitness routine.

SIDE BEND

STARTING POSITION

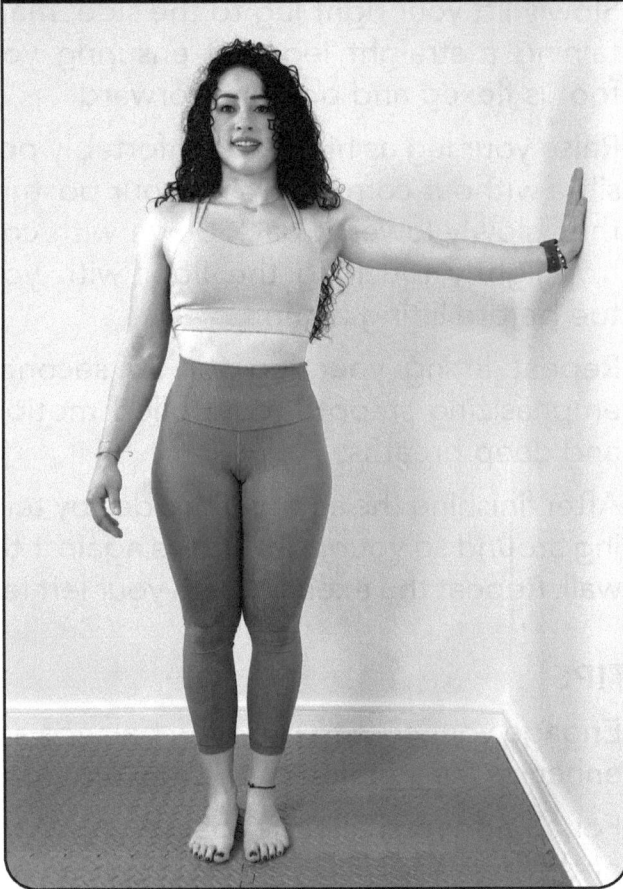

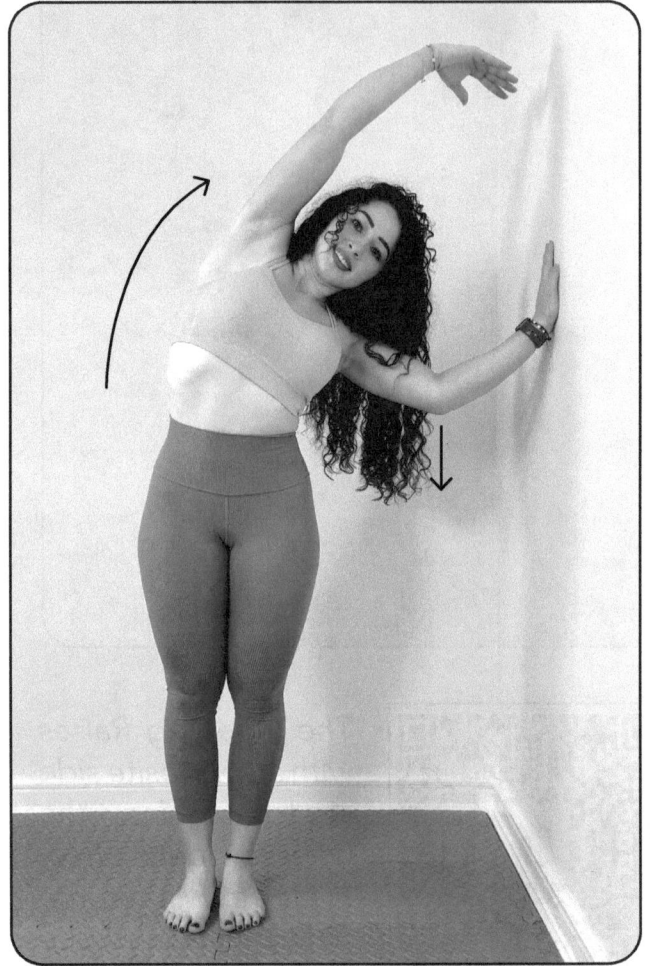

The Side Bend at the Wall is an effective stretching exercise designed to target and elongate the lateral torso muscles, including the obliques and latissimus dorsi, as well as enhancing intercostal flexibility. This exercise aids in increasing the lateral range of motion, releasing built-up tension along the sides of the body, and promoting better postural alignment by encouraging a balanced stretch on both sides of the torso.

INSTRUCTIONS

1. Stand with your left side facing the wall, feet shoulder-width apart for stability. Place your left hand on the wall at shoulder height.

2. Slowly slide your left hand down the wall while simultaneously reaching your right arm over your head towards the left side. Keep your hips and shoulders aligned, avoiding any forward or backward leaning.

3. As you reach the maximum point of your side bend, press gently into the wall with your left hand for added support and deepen the stretch. Ensure your head is in a neutral position, aligned with your spine.

4. Maintain the side bend for 20-30 seconds, focusing on deep, steady breaths to enhance the stretch along your right side. Feel the elongation from your right hip through the side of your torso and up to your right fingertips.

5. Gently come back to the starting position and repeat the stretch on the opposite side, using your right hand on the wall and bending to your right while reaching over with your left arm.

✗ MISTAKES TO AVOID

- **Overstretching:** Avoid pushing the stretch to the point of pain. The intensity should be comfortable and sustainable.

- **Twisting the Torso:** Keep your chest and hips facing forward to prevent twisting, ensuring the stretch focuses on the lateral side.

- **Neglecting Arm Extension:** Ensure the overhead arm remains straight and engaged, maintaining a constant extension to enhance the stretch along your side.

SPINE ROTATION

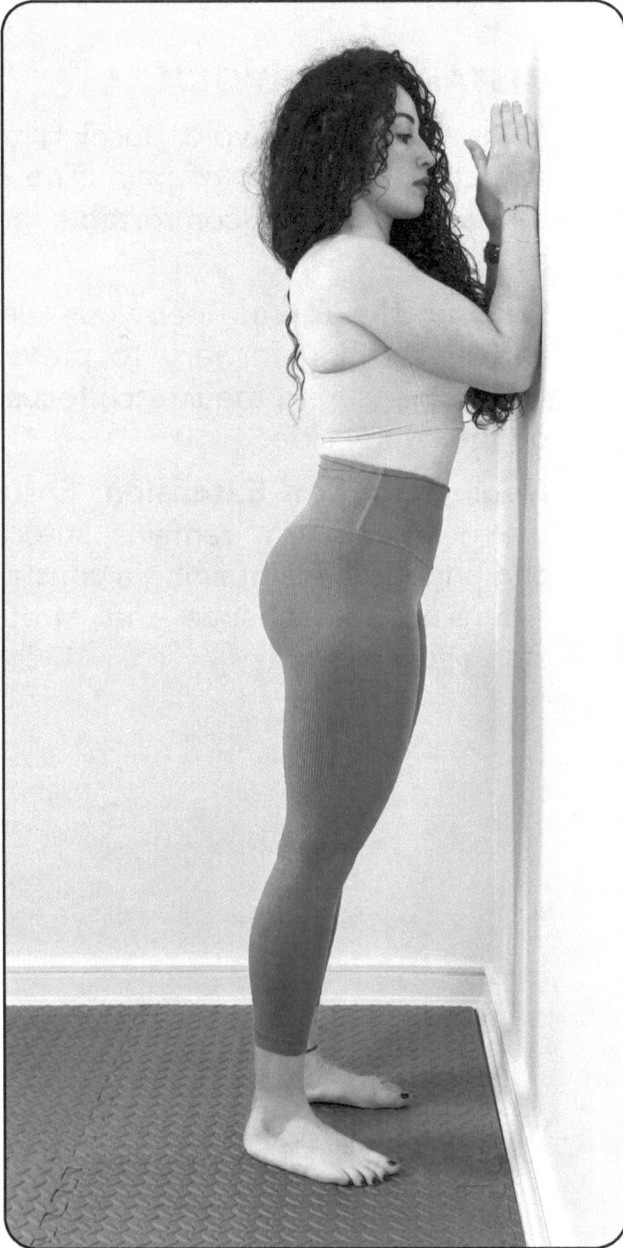

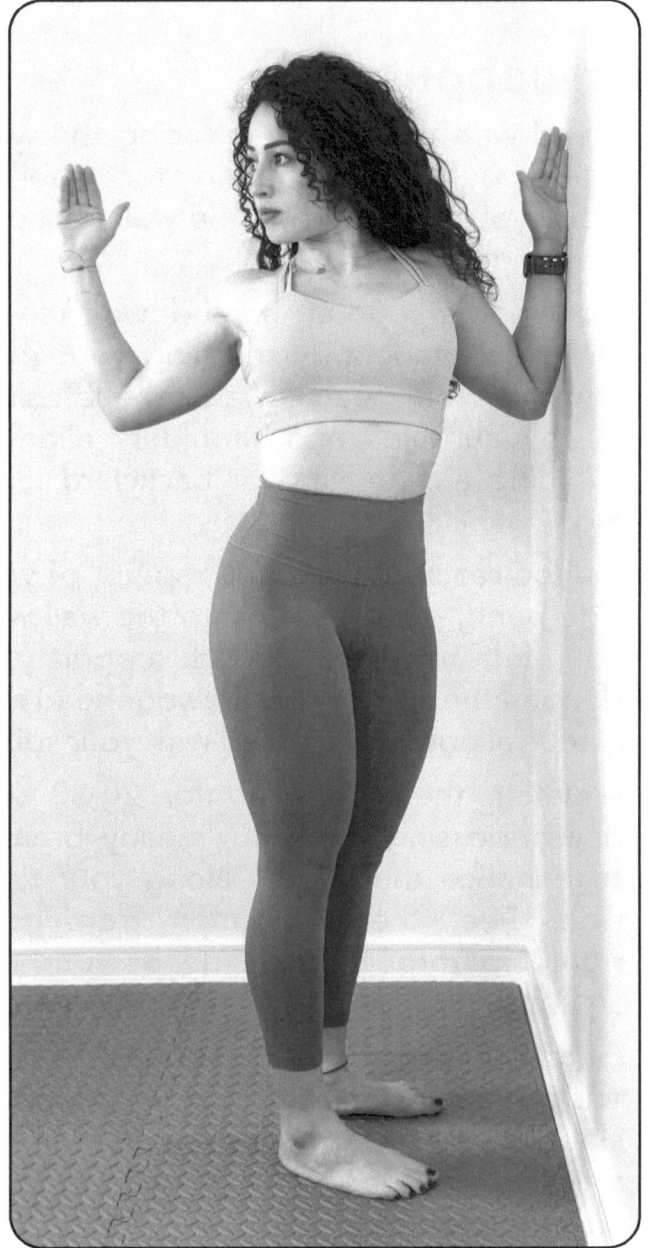

The Spine Rotation is an exercise designed to improve spinal mobility, increase thoracic rotation, and enhance overall flexibility. This movement also engages the core muscles, aiding in the stabilization of the spine during rotation. By performing this exercise against a wall, individuals can ensure proper form and alignment, maximizing the benefits of the movement for improved posture and reduced tension in the back.

INSTRUCTIONS

1. Start by standing about one foot away from the wall, with your feet hip-width apart.
2. Place the side of your forearms against the wall, elbows bent, emulating a plank position. This is your starting position.
3. Keep your lower body steady and facing forward.
4. While keeping one arm planted firmly on the wall, rotate your torso to the opposite side. Follow the rotation with your neck and gaze, ensuring a full range of motion.
5. Hold the rotated position for a moment to deepen the stretch, then slowly return to the starting position.
6. Repeat the rotation on the other side.
7. Aim for 30 seconds, focusing on smooth, controlled movements.

✓ TIPS

- Maintain the position of your arms consistently throughout the exercise. The rotation should originate solely from your torso.
- As you rotate to the side, open your chest and inhale deeply to enhance the stretch and promote relaxation. Exhale through your mouth as you return to the starting position.

✗ MISTAKES TO AVOID

- **Losing Lower Body Stability:** Keep your lower body, especially your hips and feet, stable and facing forward to isolate the rotation in your thoracic spine.
- **Not Following Through with Gaze:** Ensure you rotate your neck and follow your gaze along with your torso rotation. This helps to achieve a full spinal rotation and increases the stretch.
- **Avoid Dropping Shoulders:** Do not let your shoulders drop; keep them consistently engaged and aligned to maintain proper posture.
- **Overreaching:** Do not force the rotation beyond your comfortable range of motion. Gradually increase your flexibility over time with consistent practice.

WALL ANGEL

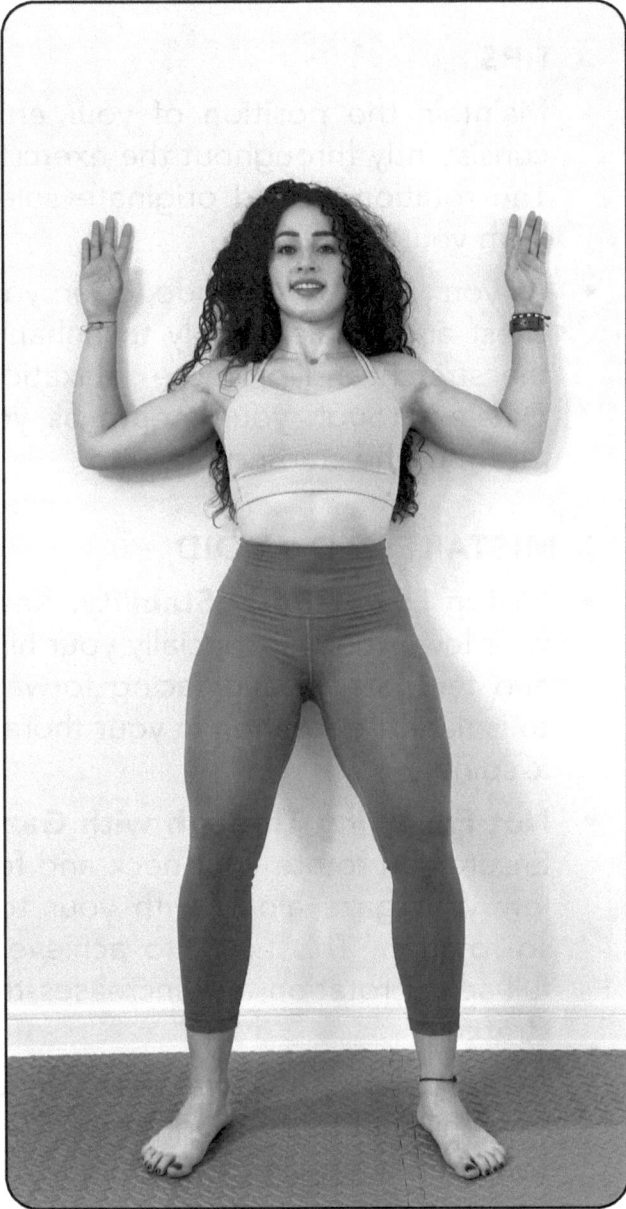 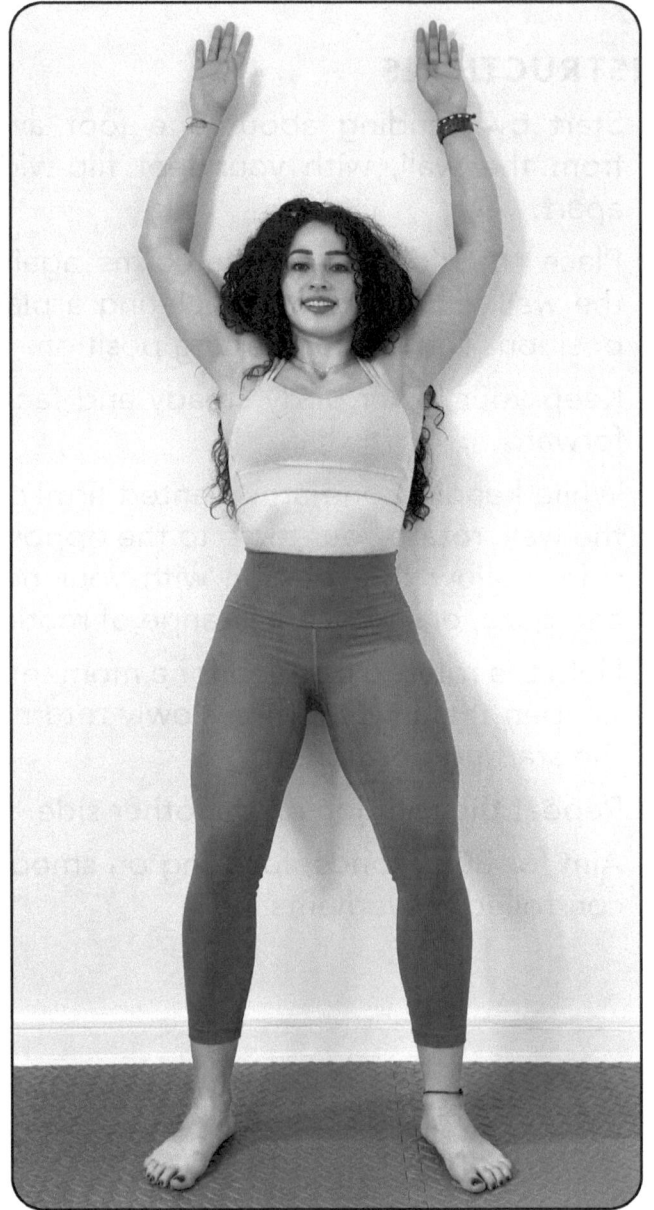

Wall Angels are effective exercises that enhance shoulder mobility, improve posture, and strengthen the upper back and scapular muscles. By performing this movement against a wall, you receive feedback on your form, ensuring proper alignment throughout the exercise. Wall Angels can help counteract the forward shoulder slump associated with prolonged sitting or computer use, making them beneficial for those suffering from back pain and looking to improve their postural awareness.

INSTRUCTIONS

1. Stand upright against the wall with feet hip-width apart, positioned slightly forward. Ensure your head, shoulders, back, and buttocks are all in contact with the wall. Adjust your chin slightly downward to allow your head to touch the wall.

2. Position your arms at shoulder level with elbows bent, forming a 'W' shape, ensuring palms face forward and the backs of your hands and arms remain in touch with the wall.

3. Slowly slide your arms up over your head. Ensure your arms, elbows, shoulders, and lower back maintain contact with the wall throughout the entire movement.

4. Gently lower your arms back to the initial 'W' shape, controlling the movement.

5. Aim to perform this exercise continuously for at least 30 seconds. Avoid pushing beyond your limits; if you start to compromise your form because of tiredness, stop the set and take a moment to recover. Preserving the integrity of your form is key to getting the full benefits of the exercise.

✓ TIP

- If sliding your arms straight up is uncomfortable, adjust the angles by extending them out to the side, forming a wide 'V' shape, while ensuring the backs of your hands and arms maintain contact with the wall. The specific shape your arms create is less important than maintaining symmetry and consistent wall contact.

✗ MISTAKES TO AVOID

- **Losing Contact:** Avoid allowing any part of your arms or back to lose contact with the wall. If this occurs, adjust your range of motion until you can maintain constant contact.

- **Forcing the Movement:** Never force your arms into an uncomfortable position. Remain within a range that feels comfortable for you.

- **Arching the Back:** Prevent your lower back from curving off the wall by activating your core muscles.

- **Improper Chin Position:** Avoid jutting your chin forward or tucking it excessively. A minimal tuck maintains alignment and supports correct posture.

SCARECROW ROTATION

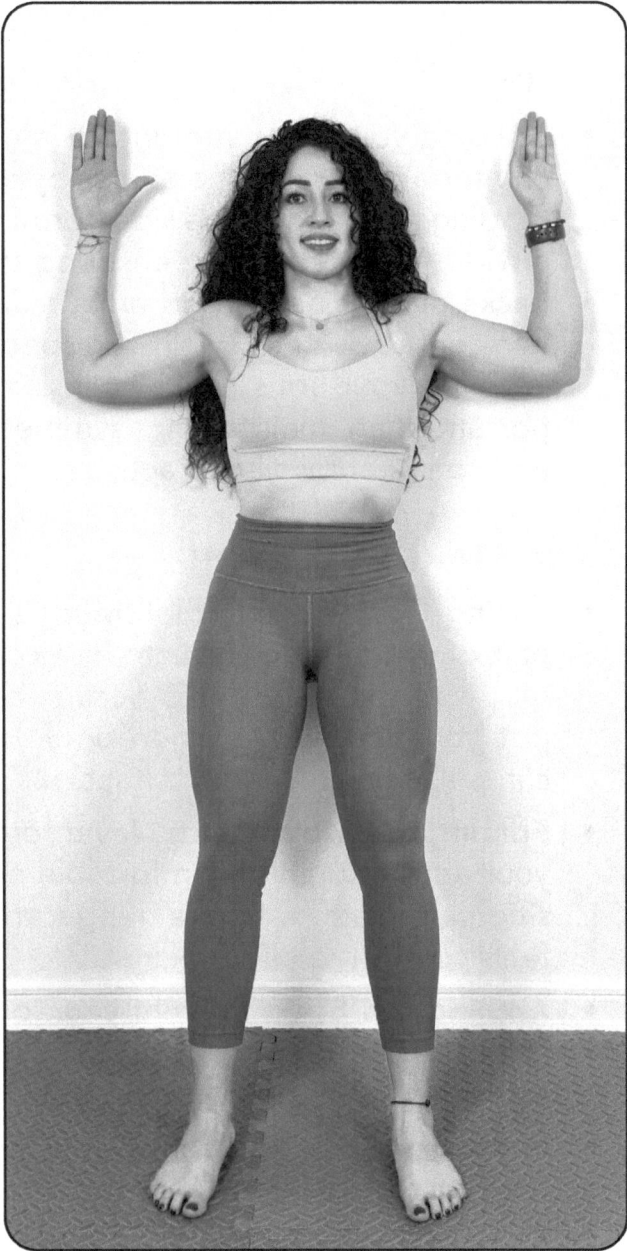

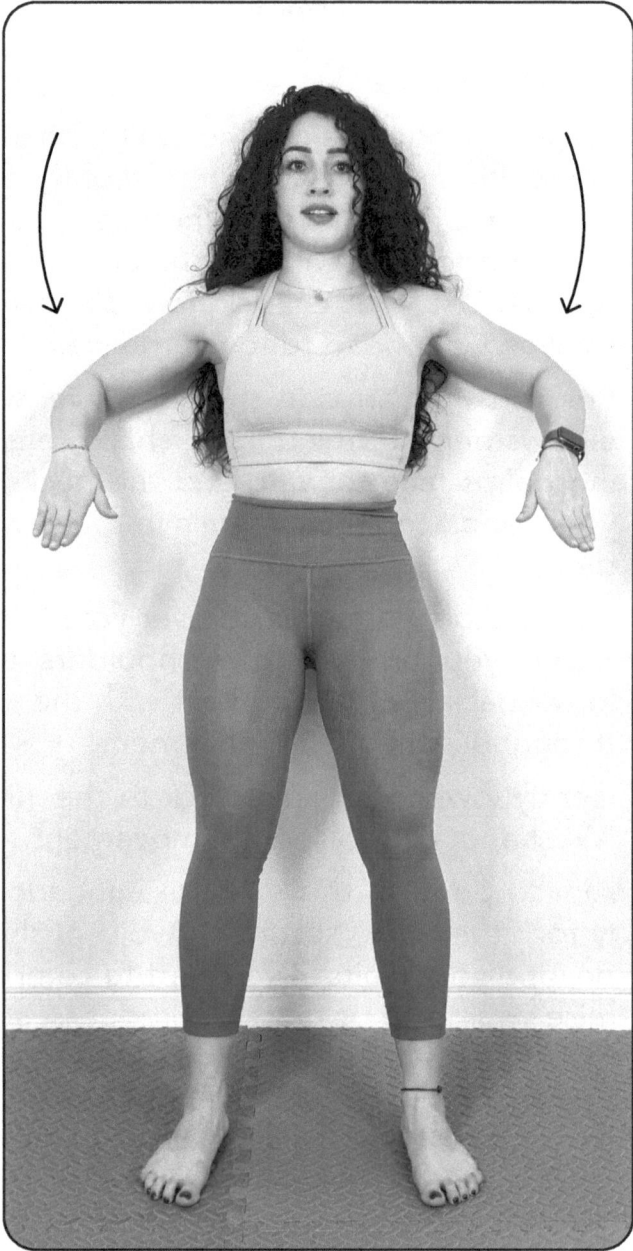

The Scarecrow Rotation is an effective exercise that targets the shoulders, particularly focusing on the rotator cuff muscles. This exercise enhances shoulder mobility and stability, crucial for various upper body movements and injury prevention. By performing this exercise against a wall, it ensures proper alignment and feedback, encouraging correct posture throughout the motion.

INSTRUCTIONS

1. Stand with your back against the wall, feet shoulder-width apart. Ensure that your head, shoulders, and lower back maintain contact with the wall throughout the exercise.

2. Raise your arms to the sides to form a 90-degree angle at your elbows, with your upper arms parallel to the floor and your forearms pointing upward, palms facing forward.

3. Rotate your upper arms forward to lower your fingertips toward the floor as far as your range of motion allows. Hold this position for one or two seconds.

4. Reverse the motion by rotating your arms at the shoulders to lift your fingertips back up, returning to the starting position.

5. Continue this movement for 30 seconds, focusing on controlled and deliberate motions to effectively engage your shoulder muscles.

✓ TIPS

- Incorporate deep, steady breathing to help maintain focus and ensure a rhythmic pace throughout the exercise.

- Enhance the exercise's challenge by using light dumbbells after mastering the basic movement. This addition will further engage and strengthen your shoulders.

✗ MISTAKES TO AVOID

- **Losing Wall Contact:** Ensure your head, shoulders, and upper arms remain in contact with the wall throughout the exercise to maintain proper alignment and effectiveness.

- **Rushing the Movements:** Rushing can lead to a loss of form and less effective muscle engagement. Take the time to execute each rotation fully, maintaining control and precision to maximize benefits.

- **Over-rotating:** Avoid rotating your arms beyond your comfortable range of motion. Excessive rotation can strain the shoulder joint. Aim for controlled, deliberate movements within your mobility limits.

KNEELING THORACIC ROTATION

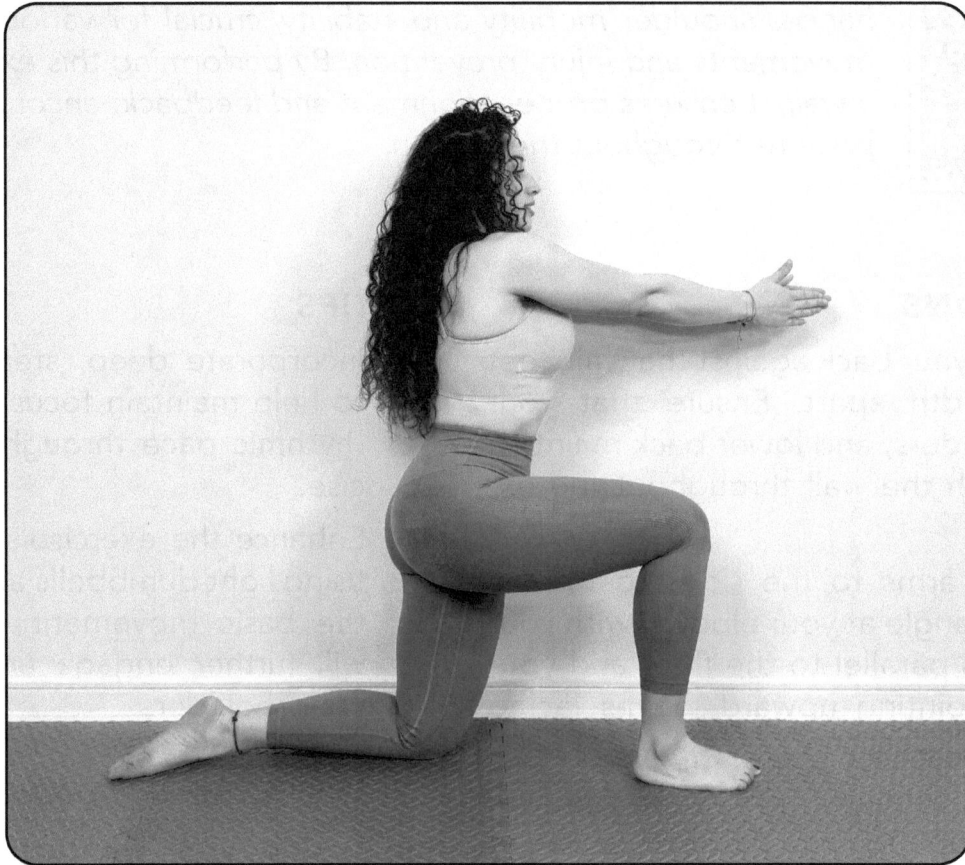

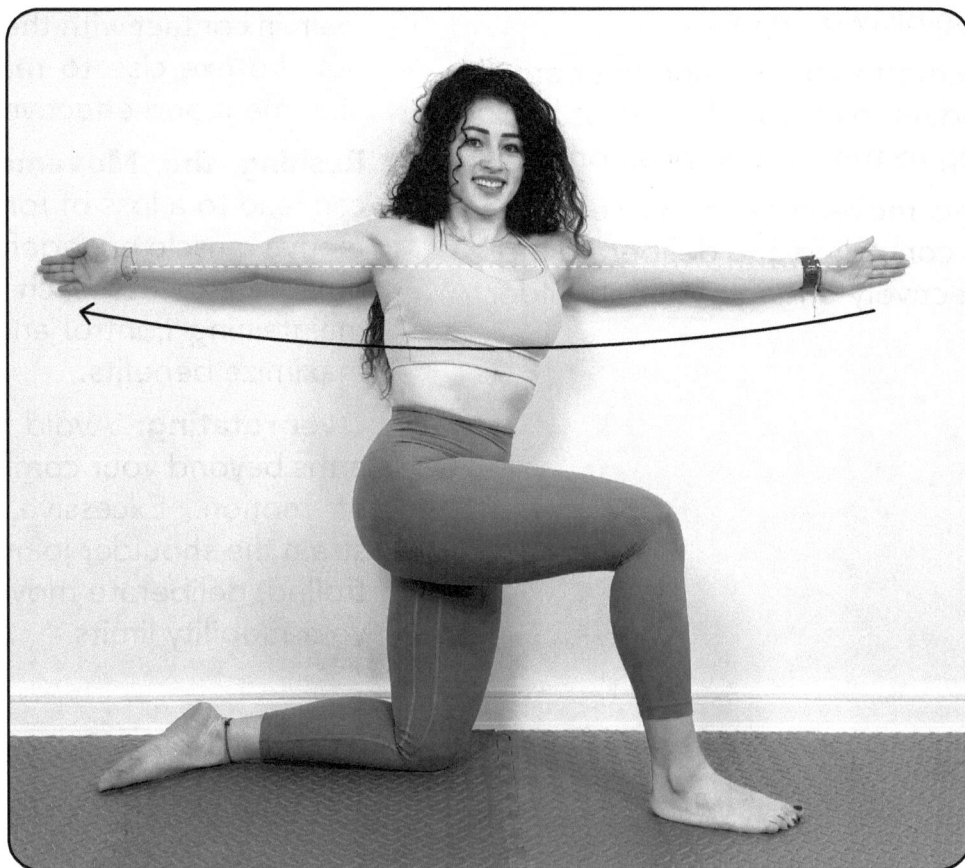

The Kneeling Thoracic Rotation exercise is designed to enhance thoracic mobility, an essential aspect of spinal health. This exercise targets the midsection of the spine, promoting flexibility, reducing stiffness, and improving posture. Performing this rotation can also alleviate tension in the upper back and neck, making it ideal for individuals who spend long hours sitting or engaging in repetitive movements.

INSTRUCTIONS

1. Start by kneeling beside the wall, positioning the leg that's farthest from the wall forward, creating 90-degree angles at both knees.

2. Press your palms together and extend your arms forward, ensuring the back of the arm closest to the wall makes contact with it at shoulder height.

3. Keep your hips stable, rotate your torso, and extend the arm farthest from the wall out to the side and then behind you, aiming to touch the wall with the back of your hand. Extend your arm towards the wall as much as possible while maintaining shoulder alignment.

4. Slowly return your arm to the starting position in a controlled manner, ensuring it stays at shoulder level.

5. Continue for 30 seconds before switching sides.

✗ MISTAKES TO AVOID

- **Arm Misalignment:** Keep the rotating arm level with the shoulders throughout the exercise to promote proper muscle engagement.

- **Rotating the Lower Body:** Keep your pelvis stable throughout the exercise to isolate the thoracic rotation and enhance the stretch's effectiveness.

- **Overstretching:** Use the wall as a guide to maintain form, not a target to forcibly reach. Keep one side in contact while rotating, but avoid extending beyond your comfortable range of motion. Flexibility will improve naturally over time with consistent practice.

- **Avoid Wrist Twisting:** While reaching for the wall, resist the urge to twist your wrist for extra length. Such twisting deviates from the exercise's objective and could introduce undue strain. Maintain alignment through your arm and wrist, focusing on proper form to ensure safe and effective rotation.

WALL COBRA

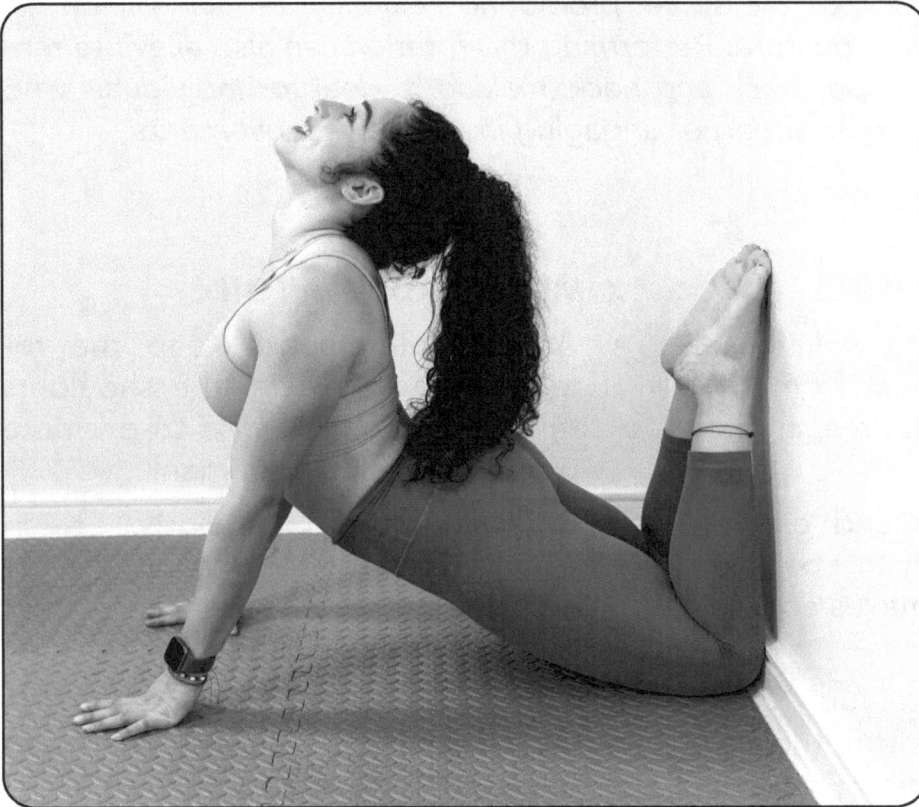

The Wall Cobra is a variation of the yoga pose that combines the benefits of the traditional cobra pose with wall support to enhance spinal extension and flexibility. This pose provides a deep stretch on your lower back, shoulders and neck.

INSTRUCTIONS

1. Begin in a prone position with your knees at the wall's base and your shins extending vertically up the wall. Your thighs, abdomen, and chest should be in contact with the floor. Position your palms flat on the floor right beneath your shoulders, with your elbows bending close to your torso.

2. Inhale deeply, and while exhaling, firmly press into your palms to elevate your chest off the ground. Engage your knees by pressing them down, subtly tuck your pubic bone towards your navel to elongate your spine. As you lift, widen your chest and spread your collarbones apart.

3. Gently extend your neck, tilting your head back in the direction of your feet, but ensure to keep the movement gentle to avoid straining. Stay in this position for a few breaths, focusing on a steady, controlled breath.

4. To exit the pose, slowly return your gaze forward to a neutral position and gradually bend your elbows, lowering your upper body back to the floor with care and control.

✓ TIP

• For a deeper stretch, gently press your pelvis forward.

✗ MISTAKE TO AVOID

• **Losing Leg Engagement:** Continuously press your shins into the wall and your knees down to the floor to stabilize the pose and enhance the stretch in your lower back.

SPINE EXTENSION

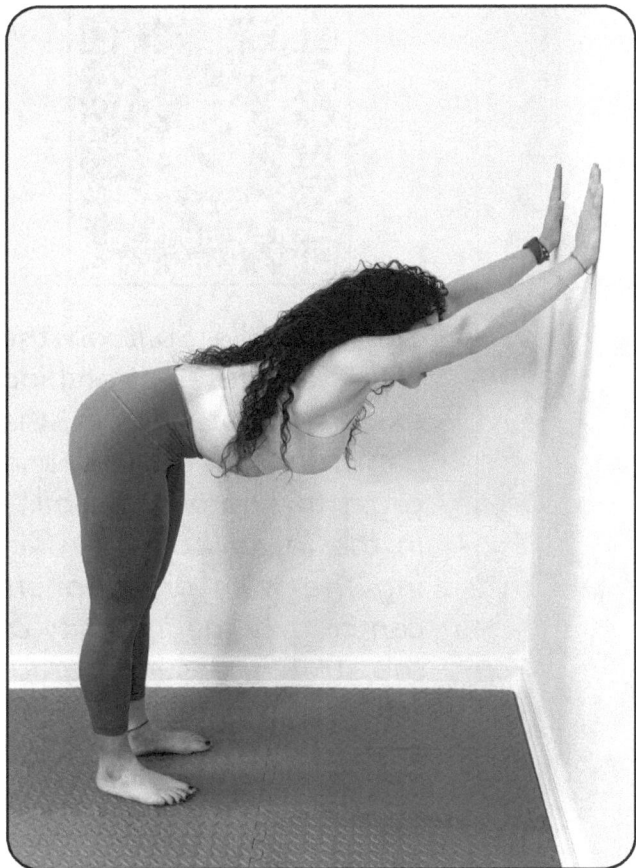

The Spine Extension on the wall is an exercise aimed at improving spinal flexibility and reinforcing the core and spinal support muscles. This activity focuses on gentle spinal extension rather than bending, encouraging the spine to elongate and the abdominal muscles to stretch and relax. It counteracts the compression effects daily sitting can have on the spine, promoting better posture and spinal alignment.

INSTRUCTIONS

1. Stand facing the wall with your feet shoulder-width apart for stability. Extend your arms and place your hands on the wall at shoulder height.

2. Gently lean into the wall, focusing on relaxing your abdominal muscles. Your torso should be parallel to the floor, creating an angle where your hips are bent at approximately 90 degrees and your legs remain straight.

3. Press your chest toward the floor, enhancing the spinal extension. Actively push through your arms keeping your elbows straight to deepen the stretch across your lats and triceps, feeling it along the sides of your back and into your arms.

4. Hold this position, concentrating on thoracic extension. Engage your abdominal muscles to prevent arching in your lower back. Breathe deeply and hold, focusing on the stretch and alignment.

✓ TIPS

- Beginners can start with hands positioned higher on the wall and the feet slightly closer to it, reducing the intensity of the lean.

- For an added challenge, carefully lift one hand off the wall at a time. This extra movement will increase the extension in your spine.

✗ MISTAKES TO AVOID

- **Avoid Overarching:** Be vigilant not to overextend or arch excessively through your lower back.

- **Neck Alignment:** Ensure your neck remains a natural extension of your spine, not craning up or tucking down, to avoid strain.

STRADDLE SPLIT

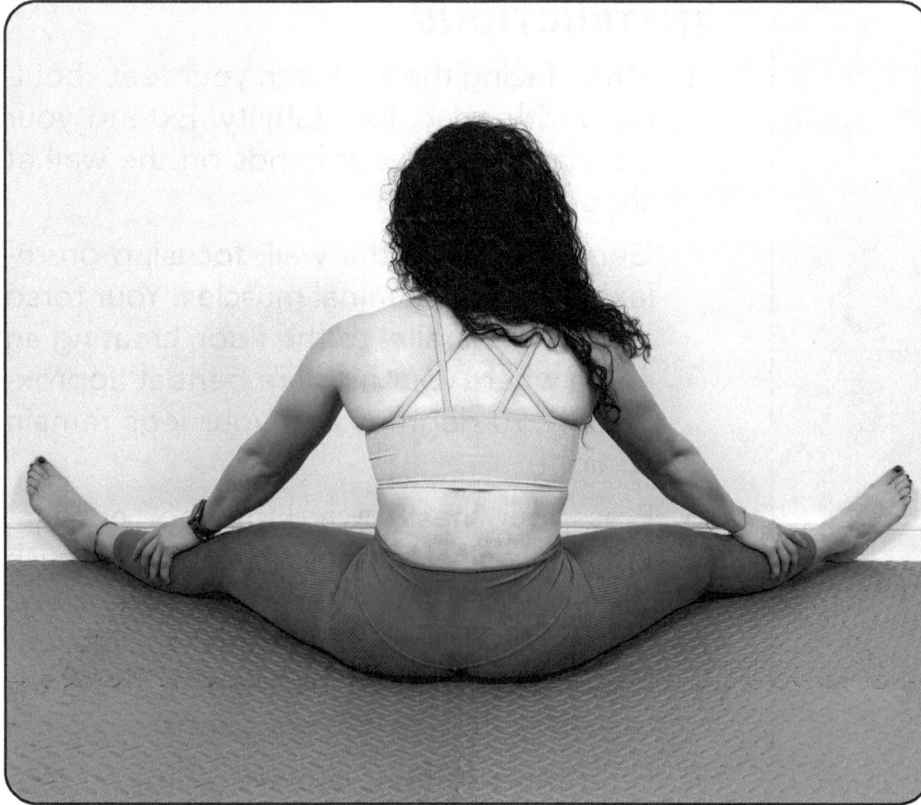

The Straddle Split on the wall is a focused stretching exercise that targets the hamstrings, adductors, and groin to improve flexibility in the lower body. By facing the wall, practitioners can control the intensity of the stretch, ensuring gradual improvement in their straddle split while maintaining alignment.

INSTRUCTIONS

1. Sit facing the wall with your legs slightly apart. Gently extend your legs to press against the wall, separating them into a wide straddle. Ensure your knees remain straight.

2. Gradually scoot forward until your pelvis is as close to the wall as comfortably achievable.

3. Place your hands on your legs or on the floor beside you for balance and support. From this position, inch your torso closer to the wall, maintaining the upright position of your spine.

4. Stay in the straddle split, focusing on relaxing your muscles and deepening the stretch with each exhalation. Aim to hold the position for several breaths or a set duration, depending on your comfort level.

5. To come out of the stretch, cautiously scoot backward, easing your legs together away from the wall.

✓ TIPS

- Ease into the stretch slowly to avoid any sudden overstretching, especially as you move closer to the wall.

- Utilize deep, measured breaths to enhance relaxation and facilitate the stretch.

✗ MISTAKES TO AVOID

- **Overstretching:** Never push yourself into pain or discomfort; stretching should be gradual and gentle.

- **Collapsing the Torso:** Maintain an upright torso to prevent undue pressure on the spine and to ensure an effective stretch.

STRADDLE SPLIT SIDE

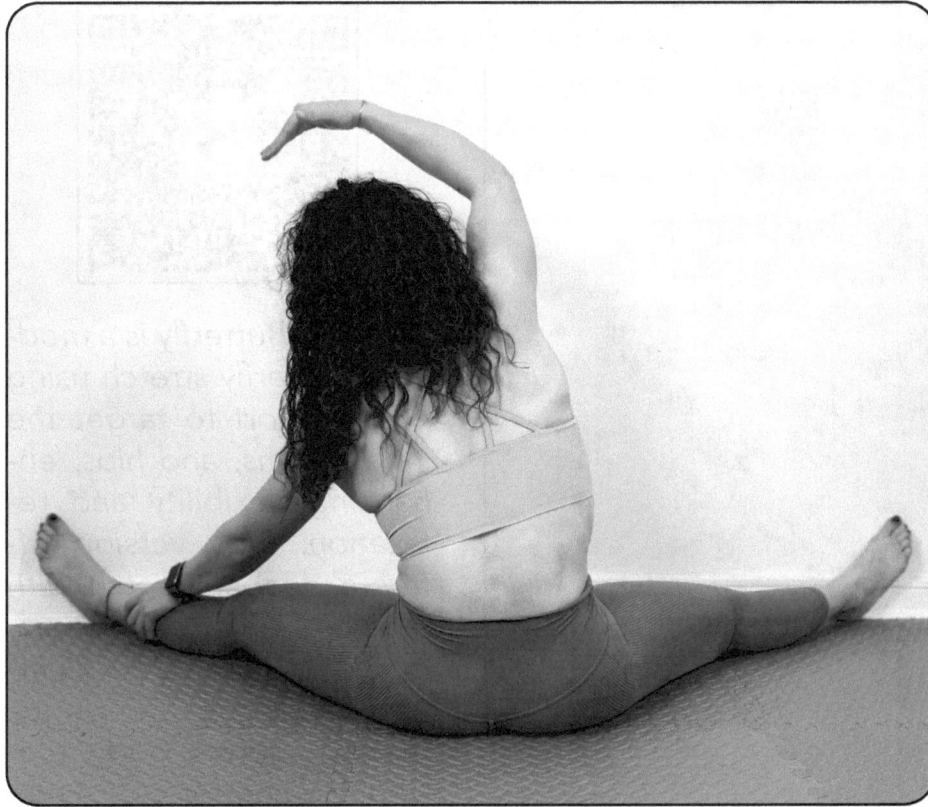

The Straddle Split Side is an enhanced version of the traditional straddle split, incorporating an upper body stretch to increase flexibility and range of motion not only in the legs but also in the torso and arms. This exercise engages the inner thighs, hamstrings, back, shoulders, and waist, providing a full-body stretch.

INSTRUCTIONS

1. Sit a comfortable distance from the wall, allowing space for a wide straddle. Gradually spread your legs into a straddle split, keeping your knees straight.

2. Gradually inch forward, allowing your torso to come closer to the wall while maintaining the straddle position. Advance until you experience a deep but comfortable stretch in your inner thighs, avoiding any discomfort or pain.

3. With your legs firmly in the straddle position, extend one arm above your head and lean to one side, creating a side stretch in your torso with the other hand resting on your leg for steadiness.

4. Maintain this side-stretching position for 15 seconds, then gently return your torso to the center before repeating the stretch on the opposite side.

✓ TIPS

- Use breath control to deepen the stretch gently, inhaling and exhaling smoothly to aid muscle relaxation and flexibility.

- Hold your neck in alignment with your spine, being cautious not to drop it when you're bending laterally.

✗ MISTAKE TO AVOID

- **Overstretching:** Avoid pushing your body into an uncomfortably wide straddle or bending excessively to the side. Always increase your range of motion gradually.

WALL BUTTERFLY

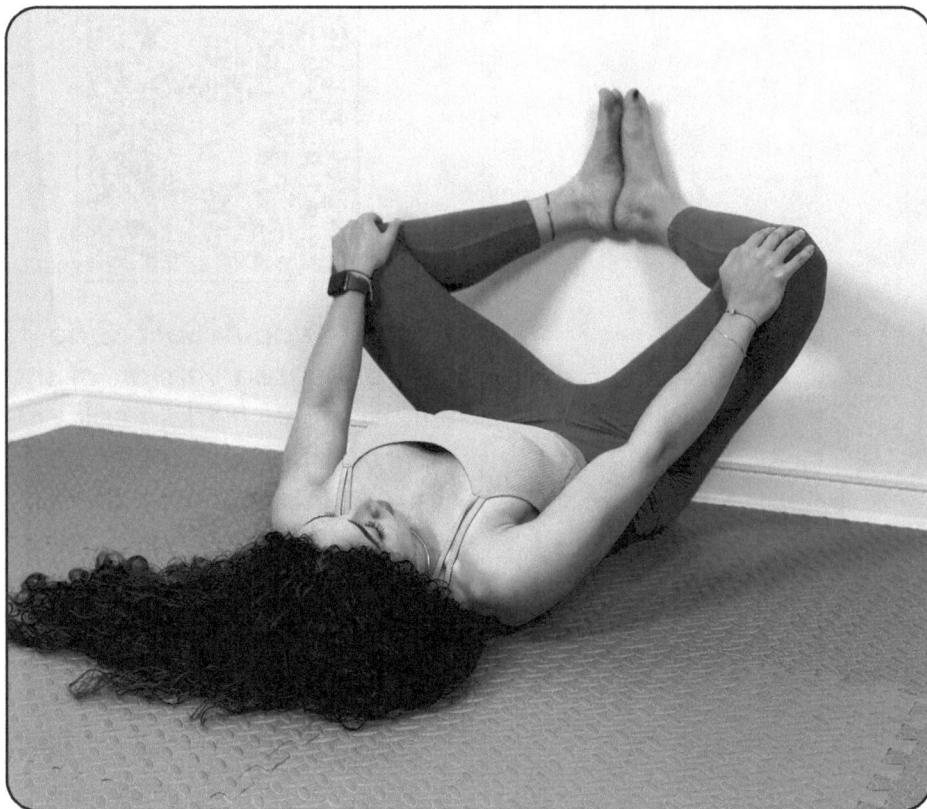

The Wall Butterfly is a modified butterfly stretch using wall support to target the inner thighs, and hips, enhancing flexibility and relaxation. This version offers a deeper stretch with reduced lower back strain, making it suitable for all fitness levels. Ideal for gently relieving lower body tension in a comfortable, lying position.

INSTRUCTIONS

1. Begin by sitting down as close to the wall as possible.

2. Gently lie on your back, placing your feet against the wall with your knees bent. Slide your buttocks closer until it touches the wall.

3. Bring the soles of your feet together using the wall for support. Allow your legs to open widely by bending your knees outward.

4. Place your hands on your side for stability or on your knees. Make sure your entire back is firmly against the floor.

5. Hold this position for at least 30 seconds, focusing on deep, steady breathing to enhance the stretch.

✓ TIP

- For a more intense stretch, use your hands to softly push your knees towards the wall. You can also increase the stretch in your lower back by gently guiding your knees towards the floor.

✗ MISTAKES TO AVOID

- **Arching Your Back:** Ensure your spine remains straight and in full contact with the floor throughout the exercise.

- **Respect Your Body's Limits:** Listen to your body and only stretch as far as feels comfortable.

CROSSED LEG STRETCH

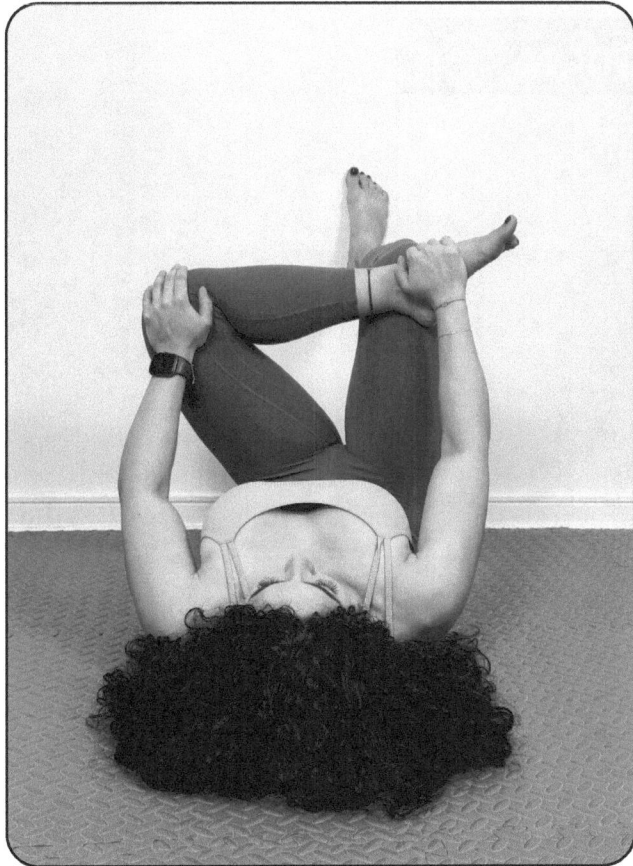

The Crossed Leg Stretch at the wall is a targeted exercise that focuses on the hips and glutes, promoting flexibility and relief in the lower back and hips. This gentle stretch is ideal for alleviating tension in the pelvic area, enhancing mobility, and can be particularly beneficial for those who experience tightness or discomfort in their lower back and hips. Furthermore, this stretch fosters better circulation in the lower body, crucial for muscle recovery and overall well-being, while also providing a therapeutic effect to reduce daily stress and enhance relaxation.

INSTRUCTIONS

1. Lie down on your back with your hips and knees bent at a 90-degree angle, feet flat against the wall.

2. Keep your right foot anchored on the wall. Carefully cross your left ankle over your right thigh, positioning it just above the right kneecap. Allow your left hip and knee to gently rotate outward.

3. Place your right hand on the elevated foot for stability. Use your left hand to gently press the left knee toward the wall, applying a soft and comfortable pressure.

4. Maintain this position for approximately 30 seconds, focusing on a gentle stretch and deep, relaxed breathing.

5. Carefully uncross your legs, placing both feet back on the wall before repeating the stretch with the right ankle crossed over the left thigh.

✓ TIP

- To modify the intensity of the stretch, you can adjust how close your hips are to the wall; moving closer will intensify the stretch, whereas moving further away will lessen it.

✗ MISTAKE TO AVOID

- **Overpressing the Knee:** Avoid applying excessive force to your knee. Exert gentle pressure to encourage the stretch without causing strain.

L LEG STRETCHING

STARTING POSITION

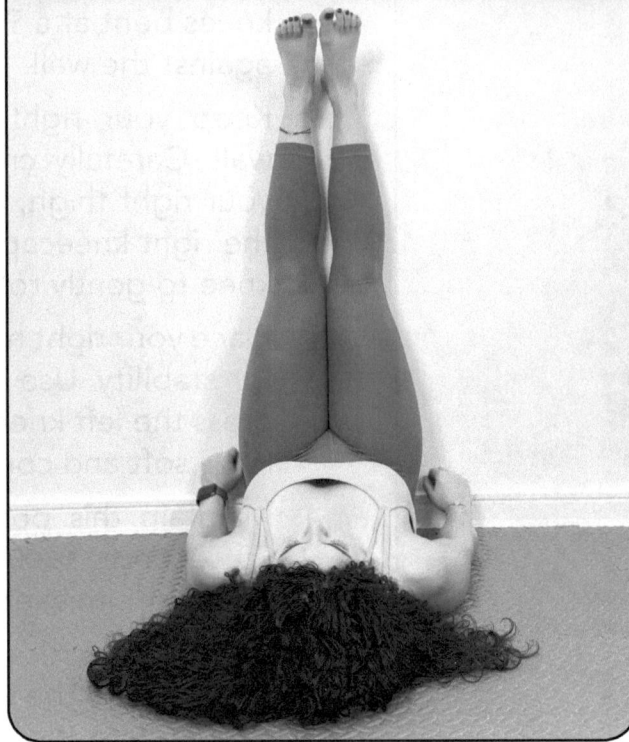

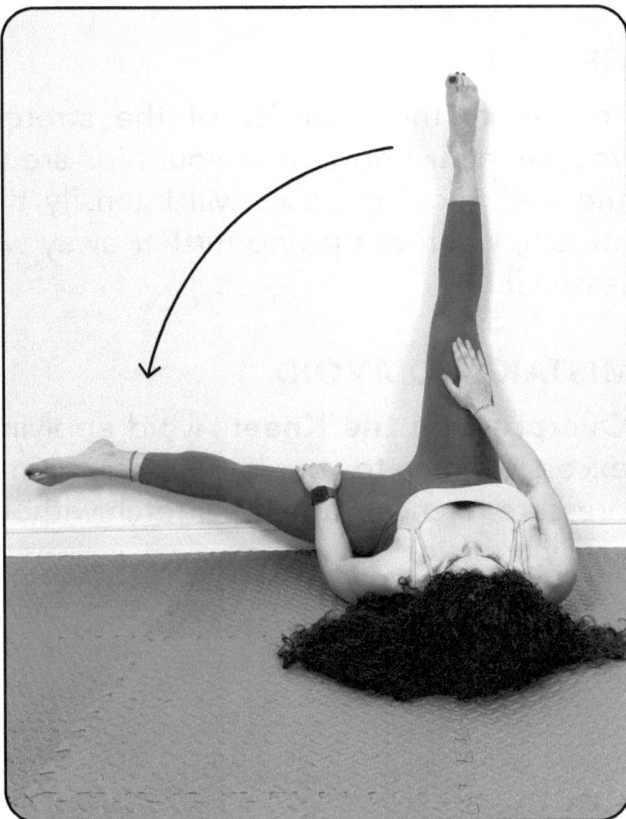

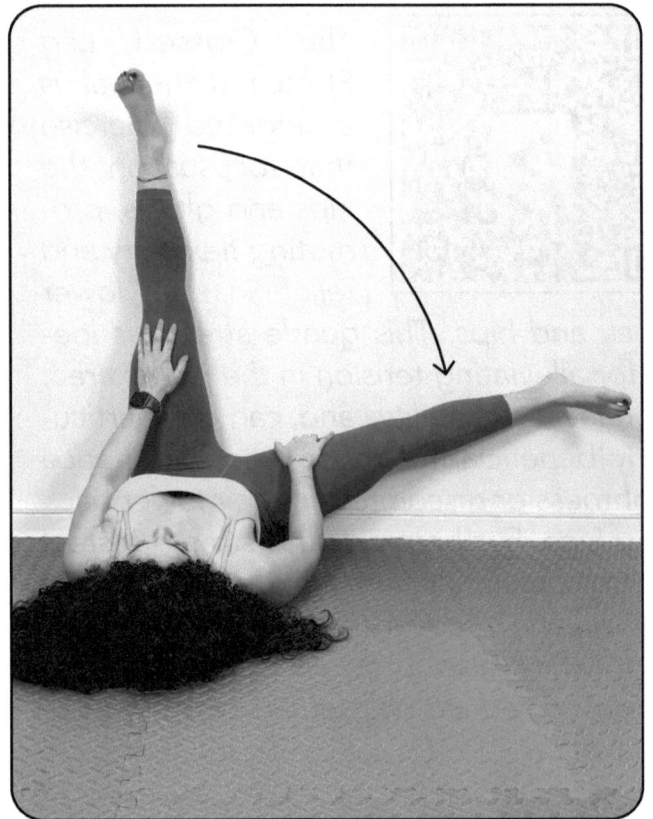

The Wall L Leg Stretching is an effective lower-body exercise designed to target the inner thighs, hamstrings, and groin area, enhancing flexibility and circulation in these key muscle groups. By utilizing the wall for support, this stretch allows for a focused and controlled approach to improving leg flexibility, which is beneficial for various physical activities and overall mobility.

INSTRUCTIONS

1. Lie on your back on the floor with your buttocks as close to the wall as possible. Extend your legs upward, pressing them gently against the wall.

2. Carefully open one leg out to the side, keeping the other leg straight against the wall. Lower the open leg until you feel a gentle stretch through the inner thigh.

3. Rest your hands on your legs, applying a gentle pressure to the inner thigh to enhance the stretch, or simply place them at your sides for balance.

4. Maintain this position, focusing on deep and steady breaths. Hold the stretch for 20-30 seconds, allowing the tension in the inner thigh to release gradually.

5. Gently bring the leg back up to the initial position and repeat the stretch with the opposite leg.

✓ TIPS

- Focus on relaxing your hips and lower back, to maximize the effectiveness of the stretch.

- For a deeper stretch, use your hand to gently press the inner thigh of the lowered leg, increasing the stretch intensity slightly.

✗ MISTAKES TO AVOID

- **Overstretching:** Do not force your leg down further than your flexibility allows, as this can lead to muscle strains.

- **Bending the Knees:** Ensure both legs remain straight throughout the stretch. Bending the knees can reduce the effectiveness of the inner thigh stretch and may lead to incorrect posture.

- **Neglecting Breathing:** Avoid holding your breath; proper breathing helps facilitate a deeper stretch and relaxation.

SCISSORS

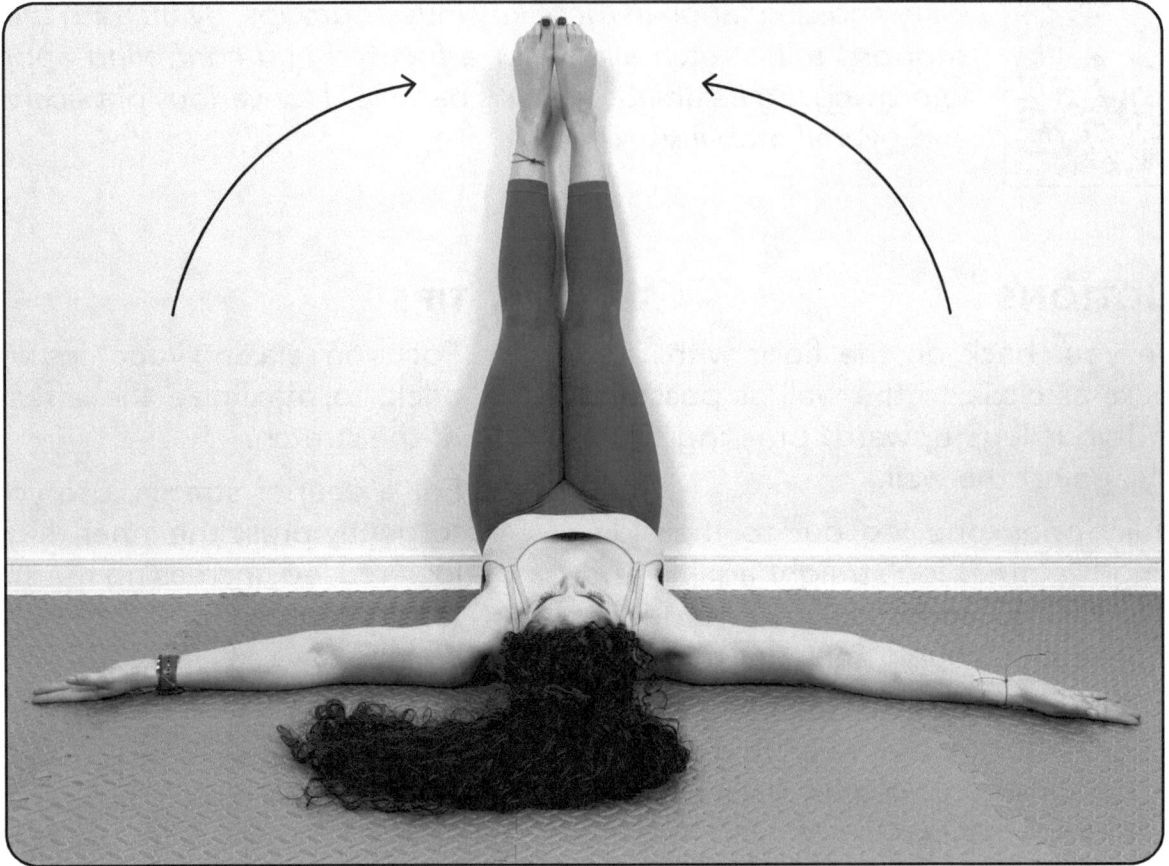

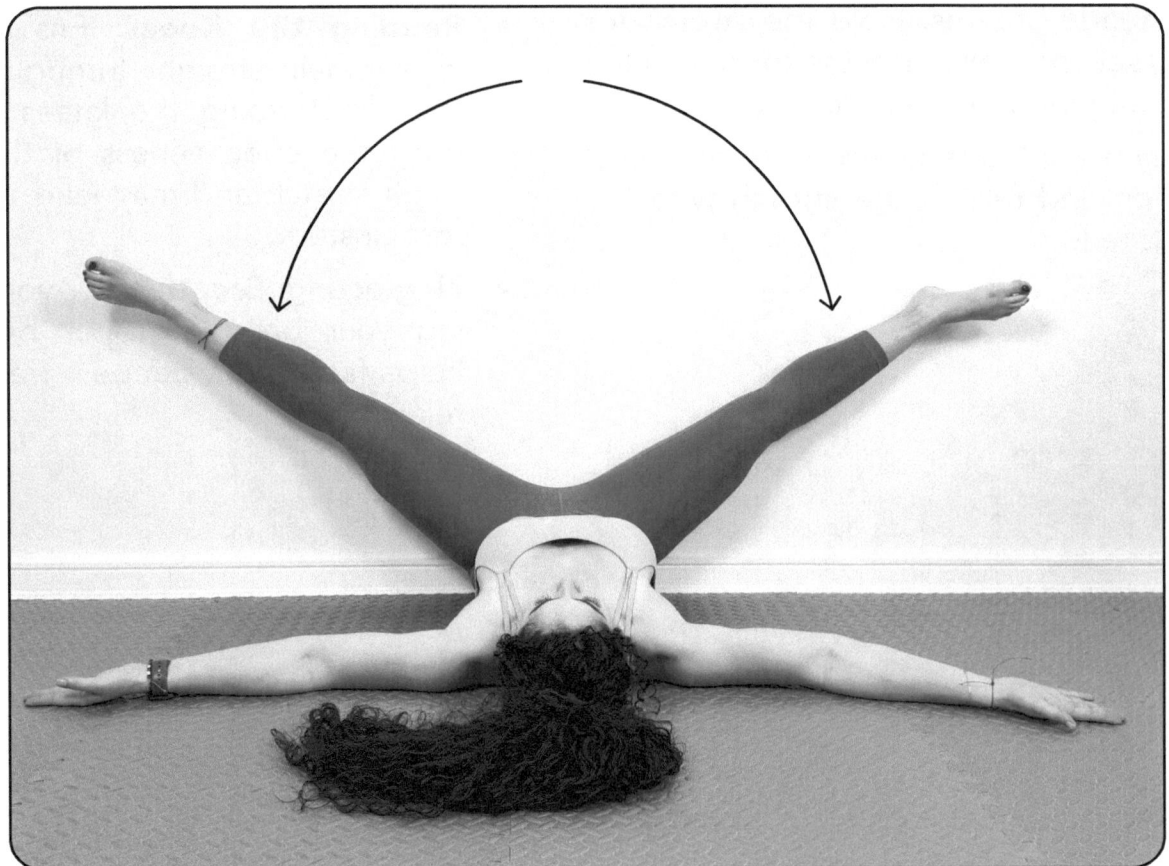

The Scissors exercise is a dynamic lower-body workout that engages your core, hips, and leg muscles, particularly targeting the inner and outer thighs. By performing this movement against the wall, you add an element of stability and resistance that can enhance muscle engagement and improve control, making it an excellent choice for both strengthening and flexibility.

INSTRUCTIONS

1. Lie on your back on the floor, facing the wall. Scoot your buttocks as close to the wall as possible and extend your legs upward, placing them against the wall.

2. Engage your core and press your lower back into the floor for stability. Gradually open your legs wide to each side, creating a 'V' shape.

3. From the 'V' shape with your legs open wide, smoothly bring both legs back up together to the initial position.

4. Ensure your legs remain straight and in contact with the wall throughout the exercise. The back of your thighs, calves, and heels should maintain contact with the wall.

5. Continue the scissor movements for a set number of repetitions or duration, focusing on maintaining form and control.

✓ TIPS

- Execute the leg movements slowly and in sync, both when opening them wide and when bringing them back together.

- Coordinate your breath with your movements—inhale while lowering and exhale while lifting—to optimize oxygen flow and muscle function.

✗ MISTAKES TO AVOID

- **Avoid Overextension:** Ensure you do not overstretch your legs throughout the exercise. Always operate within a range of motion that feels comfortable for you.

- **Avoid Rushing:** Maintain a controlled pace, ensuring your legs move together both when opening and closing. Rushing can disrupt the synchronization and reduce the effectiveness.

- **Maintain Straight Legs:** Keep both legs straight and aligned, moving in harmony to maximize the stretch's benefits and ensure even muscle engagement.

- **Ensure Posture:** Keep your lower back pressed to the floor throughout the movements to provide a stable base and prevent strain, allowing for a smoother synchronized motion of the legs.

HIP LIFTS

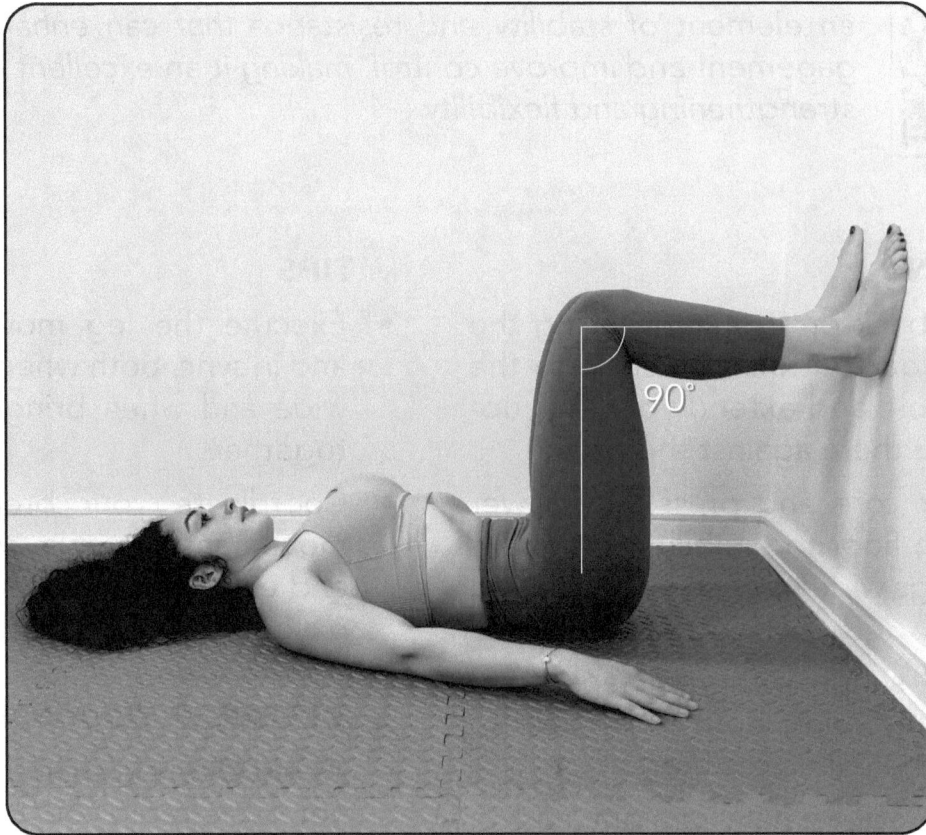

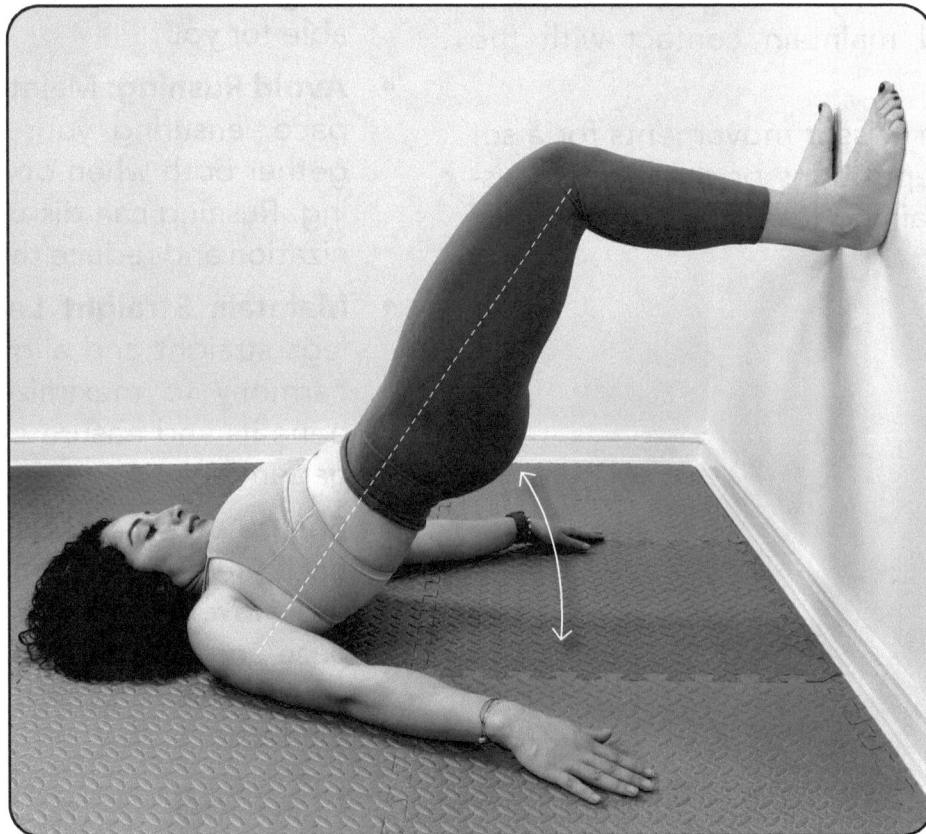

Hip Lifts against the wall are a beneficial exercise targeting the lower back, glutes, and hamstrings. Performed by lying on the back with feet pressed against the wall and knees bent, this exercise involves lifting the hips towards the ceiling to form a straight line from the shoulders to the knees. This movement strengthens the core and lower body, enhances pelvic stability, and can alleviate lower back tension.

INSTRUCTIONS

1. Begin by lying on the mat with your back pressed flat against it, gazing upwards.

2. Position your legs up against the wall with your knees creating, a 90-degree angle.

3. Place your arms by your sides, palms facing down, to aid with stability.

4. Activate your core muscles, then press your feet firmly against the wall. As you exhale, elevate your hips towards the ceiling, forming a straight line from your shoulders to your knees, engaging your glutes and hamstrings in what is known as the wall bridge position—a foundational pose for numerous wall Pilates exercises.

5. Maintain this elevated posture momentarily before gently lowering your hips to the mat on an inhale.

6. Continue this exercise for a set duration or number of repetitions.

✓ TIPS

- Keep your feet hip-width apart and parallel to each other on the wall for the best support and alignment.

- When performing the bridge position, if you see your toes extending beyond your knees, it indicates that your feet are positioned too high. Restart the exercise, ensuring your knees are bent at a 90-degree angle before performing the bridge again.

- If you experience excessive pressure on your shoulder blades, this may indicate that you are positioned too close to the wall. Readjust your starting position by moving slightly away from the wall.

- To prevent neck pain, keep your gaze towards the ceiling, not your feet.

✗ MISTAKES TO AVOID

- **Arching Your Back:** Avoid over-arching your lower back as you lift your hips. Maintain a neutral spine to prevent strain.

- **Rushing the Movements:** Perform each lift and lower with control, focusing on the quality of the movement rather than speed.

LEG CIRCLES

INSTRUCTIONS

1. Lie on your back on a mat, facing upwards, and position your legs against the wall with feet apart, pressing firmly.

2. Engage your glutes and lift your hips into a wall bridge position, keeping your core tight and back straight.

3. Extend one leg towards the ceiling, toes pointed, while the other foot remains pressed against the wall.

4. Rotate the raised leg in controlled, small circles: 5 clockwise, then 5 anti-clockwise, focusing on precision.

5. Perform for a set duration or number of repetitions, maintaining consistent breathing and proper form.

6. Lower your hips to the floor gently and switch legs to ensure balanced training.

✓ TIPS

- Maintain a firm core throughout the exercise to stabilize your bridge position and support your lower back.

- Emphasize smooth, controlled leg circles to enhance muscle activation and flexibility.

- Breathe evenly to facilitate muscle relaxation and improve the fluidity of movements.

✗ MISTAKES TO AVOID

- **Dropping the Hips:** Maintain a lifted, stable hip position throughout, using core and glute strength to support the bridge.

- **Large Circles:** Make small circles to ensure control and minimize the risk of strain.

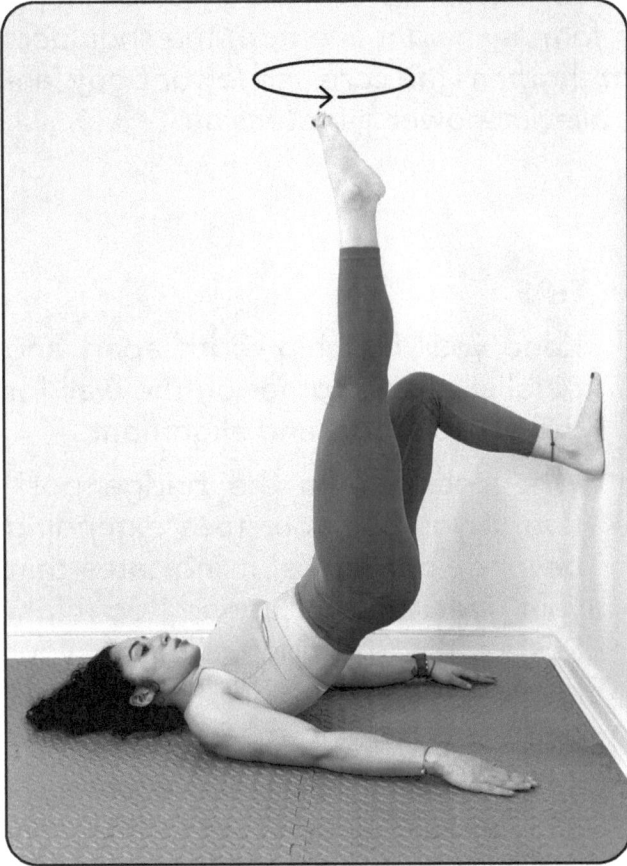

Wall Leg Circles uniquely combine the stability and core engagement of a traditional wall bridge with the mobility and flexibility benefits of leg circles. Elevating the hips and performing controlled circles with one leg targets the glutes, hamstrings, and hip flexors, while also improving leg flexibility and circulation. The synergy of bridge positioning and leg circles demands coordination and control, engaging multiple muscle groups for a holistic workout that boosts muscle strength, endurance, flexibility, and joint health.

KICKBACK HOLD

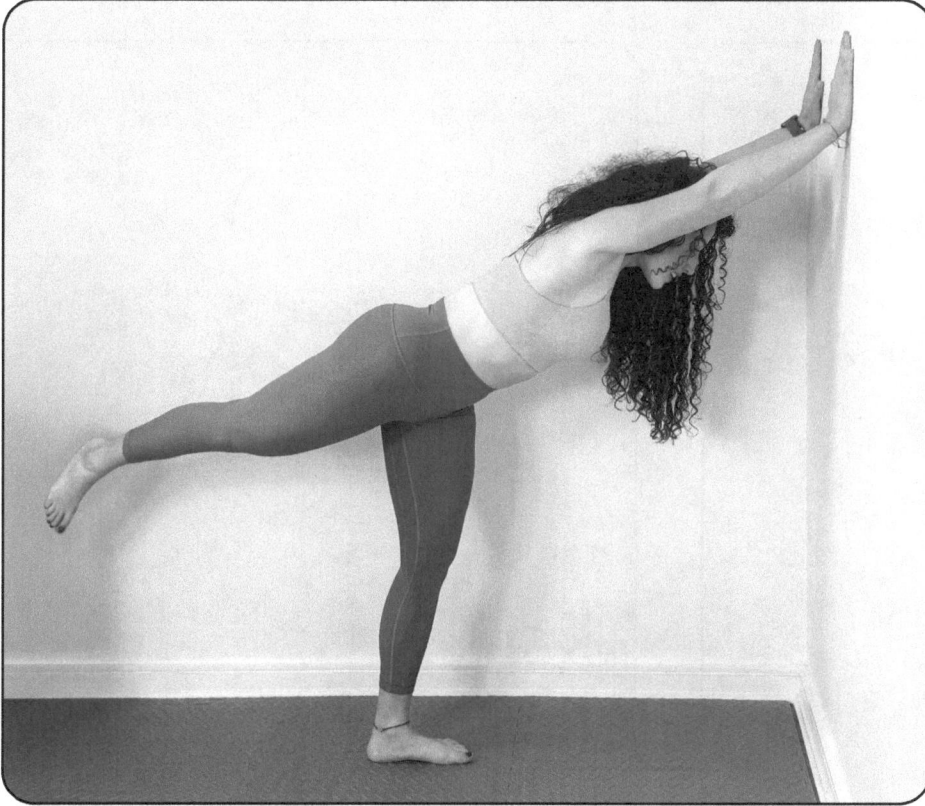

The Kickback Hold strengthens and tones the glutes using wall support for stability. This exercise emphasizes continuous muscle engagement to enhance endurance and define the lower body, also improving balance and core strength.

INSTRUCTIONS

1. Stand a large step away from the wall, facing it. Lean forward and place your palms on the wall for stability.

2. Shift your weight onto your left foot. Extend your right leg straight back as far as possible, engaging your glutes.

3. Maintain the kickback position with your right leg, ensuring your hips are even and your back remains straight. Keep your head in line with your spine.

4. Hold this position for 20-30 seconds, focusing on engaging the gluteal muscles of the extended leg and breathing naturally.

5. Gently lower your right leg, shift your weight to the right foot, and repeat the exercise with your left leg extended.

✓ TIPS

- Engage your core throughout the exercise to enhance stability and protect your lower back.

- For an added challenge, increase the hold duration or add ankle weights to intensify the muscle engagement.

✗ MISTAKES TO AVOID

- **Arching Your Back:** Keep your spine neutral to avoid strain on your lower back.

- **Bending the Extended Leg:** Keep your extended leg straight to ensure the glutes are properly engaged and the focus remains on the targeted muscle group.

SINGLE LEG LIFTS

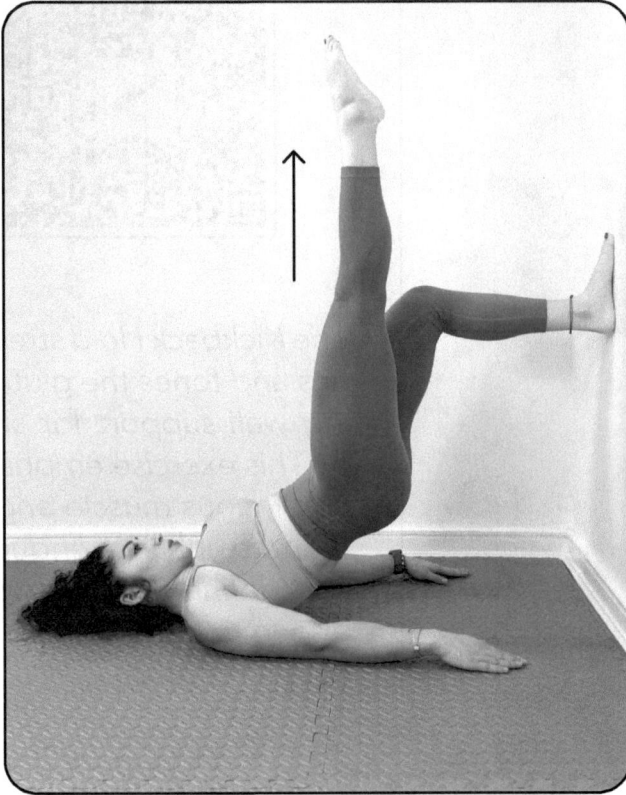
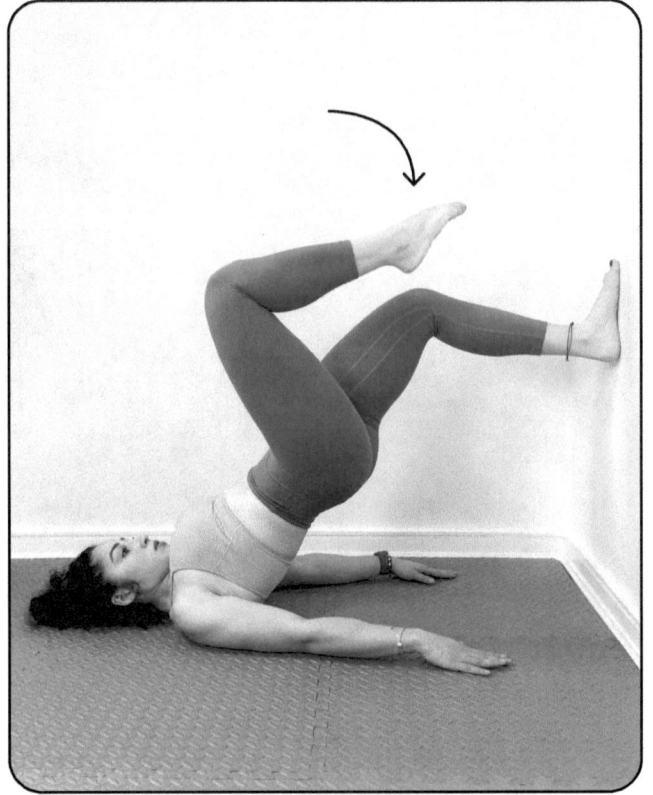

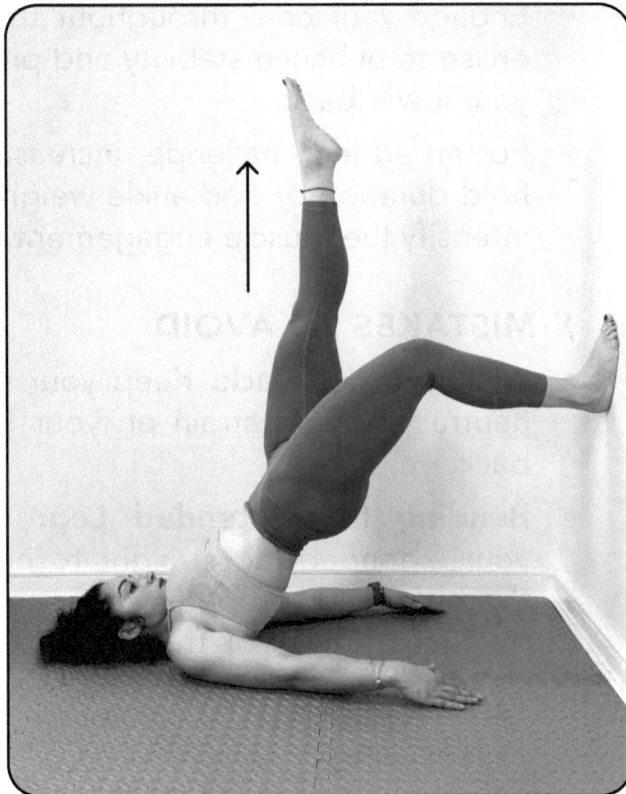
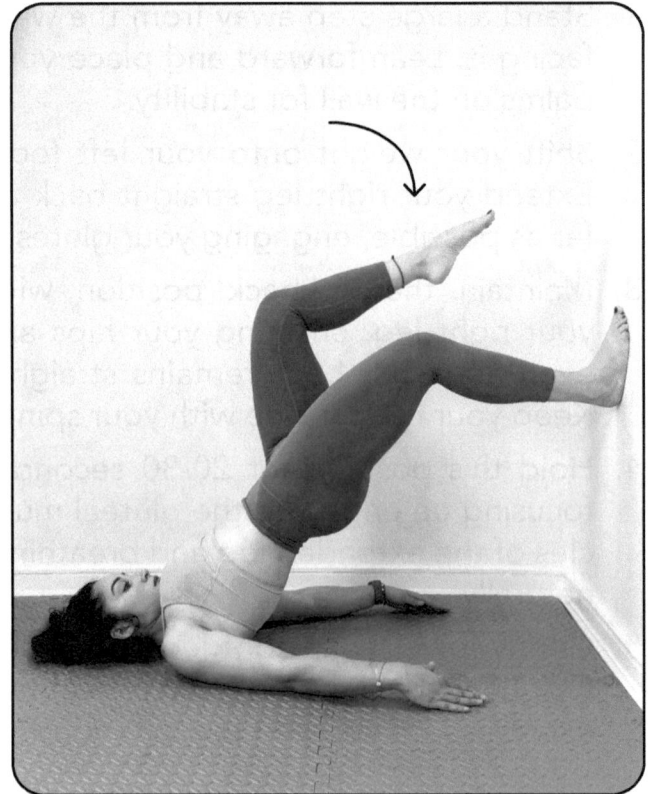

The Single Leg Lifts are a variation of the traditional bridge exercise that targets the glutes, hamstrings, and core, with an added focus on balance and unilateral strength. By lifting one leg while in the bridge position, this exercise increases the intensity, challenging stability and engaging the lower body muscles more deeply.

INSTRUCTIONS

1. Begin by lying on your back with your feet flat against the wall and your knees bent. Your arms should be flat on the floor by your sides for stability.

2. Push through your heel to lift your hips towards the ceiling, entering a bridge position with your body forming a straight line from your shoulders to your knees.

3. Steadily raise one leg off the wall, extending it straight up towards the ceiling.

4. Bend the raised leg, bringing the foot towards the wall without touching it, then straighten it back towards the ceiling.

5. Repeat this movement for a set number of repetitions or time, keeping your hips elevated and stable throughout.

6. Slowly lower the lifted leg back to the starting position on the wall and switch legs to repeat the exercise.

✓ TIPS

- Keep your core engaged and your hips lifted evenly throughout the exercise to ensure stability and effectiveness.

- Focus on smooth, controlled movements to maximize muscle engagement and prevent injury.

- Breathe consistently throughout the exercise, exhaling as you lift the leg and inhaling as you lower it.

✗ MISTAKES TO AVOID

- **Dropping the Hips:** Avoid letting your hips sag towards the floor. Keep them lifted and stable to engage the correct muscles effectively.

- **Rushing the Movements:** Perform the leg lifts and bends slowly and with control to ensure proper form and muscle engagement.

- **Losing Balance:** Ensure your supporting foot remains flat against the wall and your core is engaged to help maintain balance.

MARCHING BRIDGE

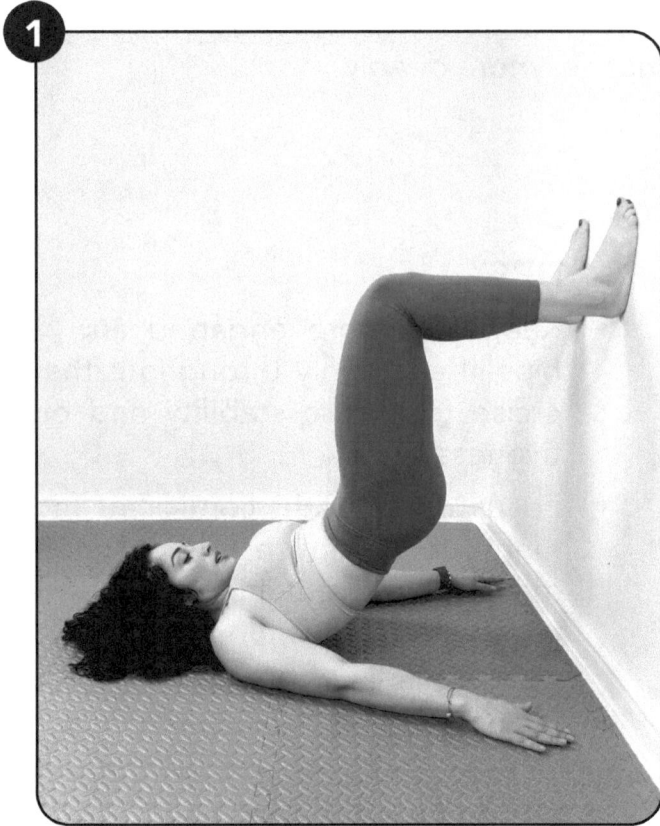

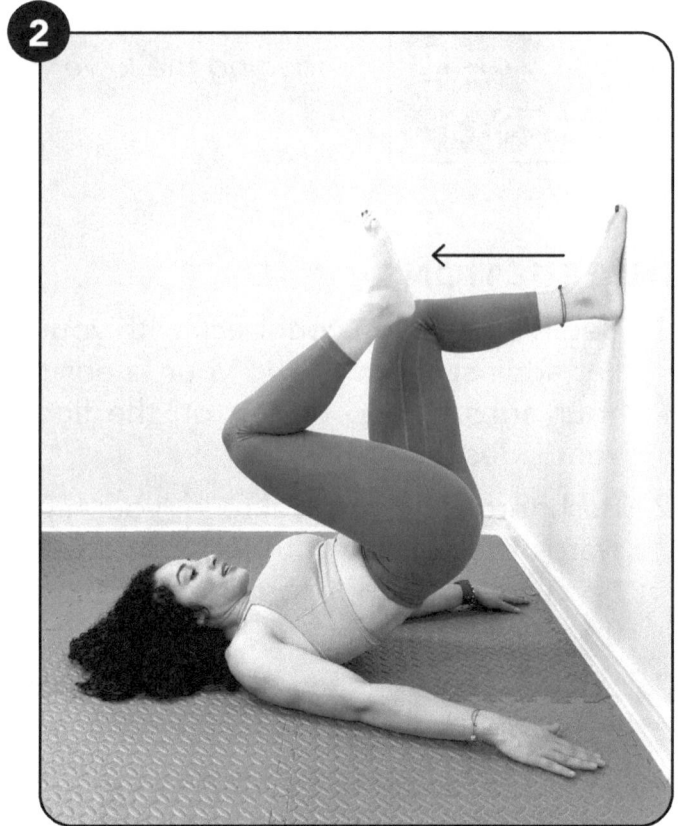

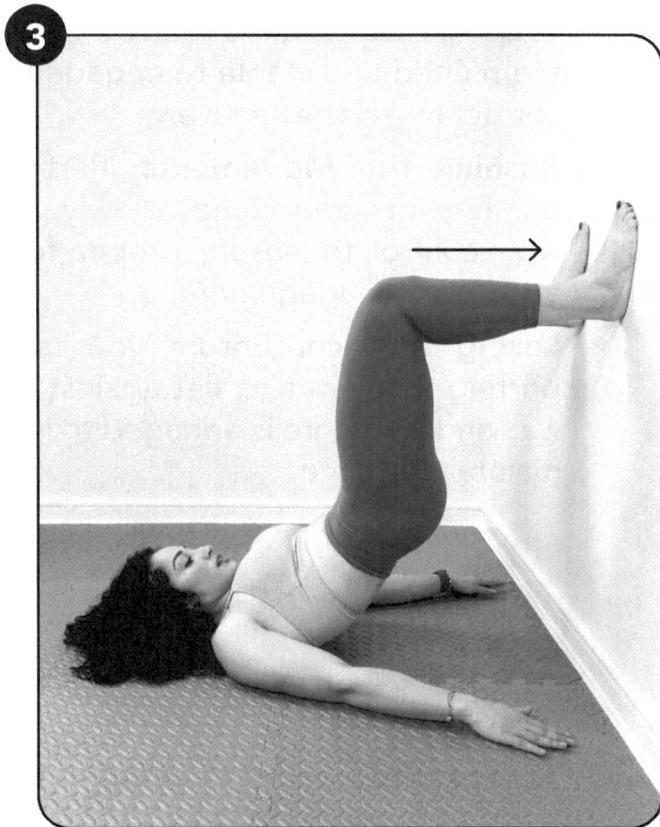

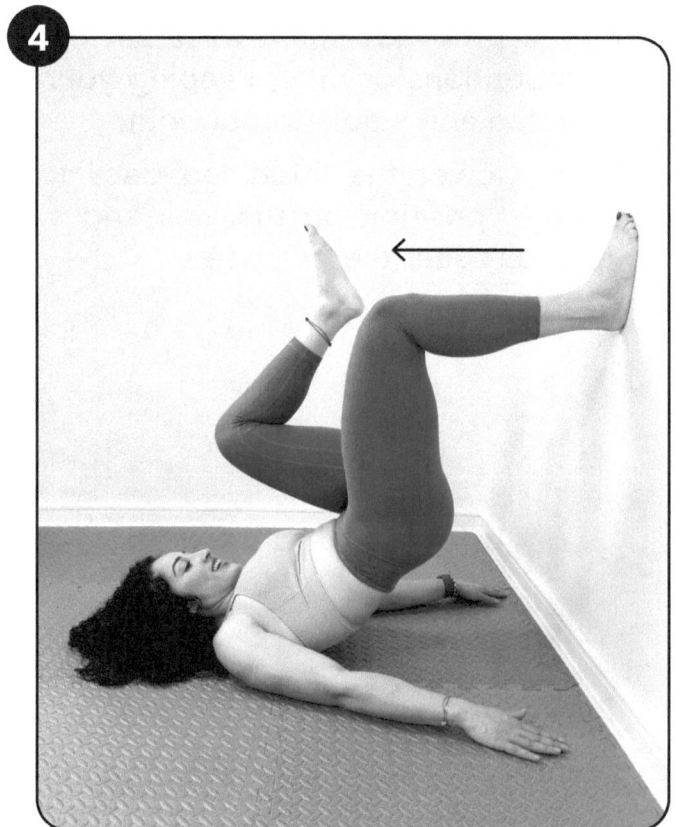

The Marching Bridge on the wall is a dynamic exercise that combines the stability of a wall-supported bridge position with the movement of marching. This exercise targets the core, glutes, and hamstrings, enhancing stability, strength, and coordination. By focusing on smooth movements rather than speed, it offers a controlled workout that emphasizes muscle engagement and balance.

INSTRUCTIONS

1. Lie on your back on the floor with your feet flat against the wall and your knees bent. Lift your hips to enter the bridge position.

2. While holding the bridge, lift one foot off the wall in a controlled marching motion, ensuring your hips remain stable.

3. Gently lower your foot back to the wall, maintaining the bridge position.

4. Lift the opposite foot, keeping your core engaged and your pelvis stable.

   Continue the exercise for a set duration or number of repetitions, focusing on the smooth execution of each march and the consistent stability of the bridge position.

✓ TIPS

- Keep your core tight throughout the exercise to support your lower back and enhance the effectiveness of the marching movement.

- Aim for smooth, controlled lifts of each foot, focusing on the stability of your hips and the engagement of your glutes and hamstrings.

- Breathe evenly throughout the exercise, coordinating your breath with each marching movement to maintain rhythm and control.

✗ MISTAKES TO AVOID

- **Rushing the March:** The focus of this exercise is on control and stability, not speed. Ensure each marching movement is deliberate and smooth.

- **Losing Core Engagement:** Maintain constant core engagement to prevent arching your back and to support your overall posture during the exercise.

- **Dropping the Hips:** Avoid letting your hips sag during the march. Keep them lifted and stable to maintain the integrity of the bridge position.

BRIDGE AND KICK

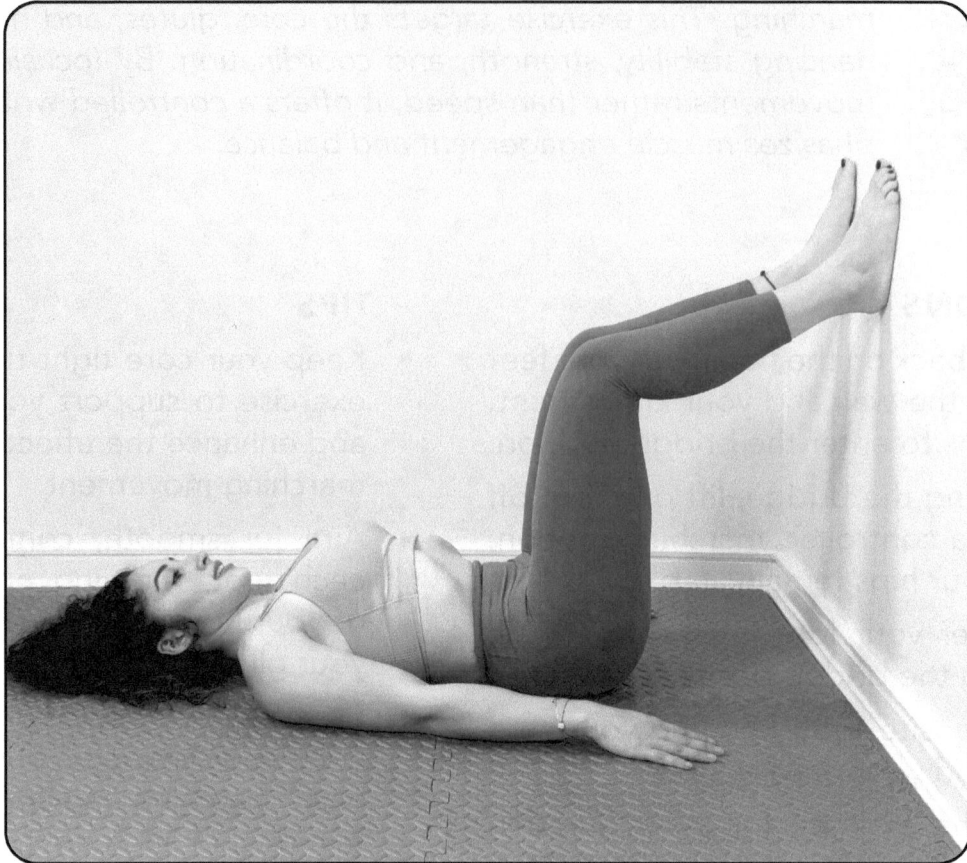

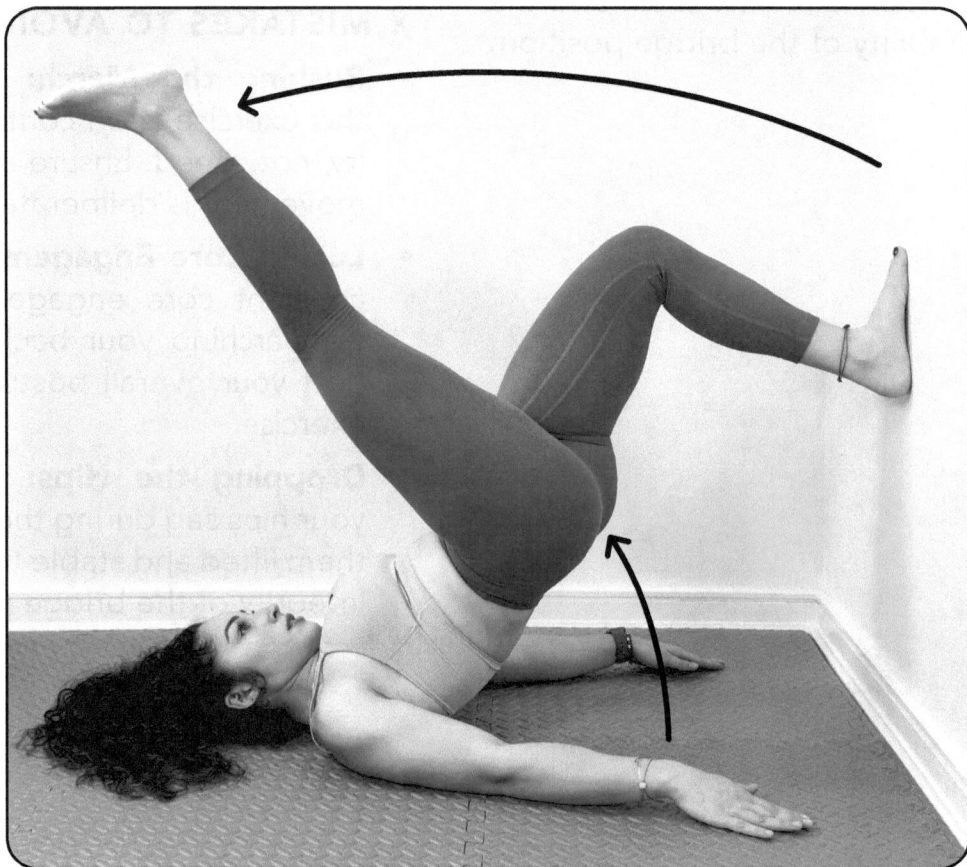

The Wall Bridge and Kick is an advanced variation of the traditional Wall Hip Lifts, incorporating a leg raise to intensify the exercise. This dynamic movement targets the glutes, hamstrings, and core while improving balance and coordination. By adding a leg kick to the bridge position, it further challenges stability and enhances muscular engagement, making it ideal for those looking to increase the difficulty of their lower body and core workout.

INSTRUCTIONS

1. Start by lying on the floor with your feet placed on the wall. Your feet can be positioned higher than your knees to provide more stability for this exercise.

2. Press one foot into the wall to lift your hips into a bridge. Simultaneously, extend your other leg in a controlled kick, aiming for straightness and distance from the wall. Keep your core and glutes engaged to maintain a straight back, ensuring proper posture and reducing the risk of strain.

3. Smoothly lower your kicking leg and hips back to the starting position, maintaining control and muscle engagement.

4. Repeat the movement, alternating legs for 30 seconds.

✓ TIPS

- Ensure your foot placement on the wall provides stable support, allowing for a solid foundation as you move into the bridge and kick.

- Gradually extend the range of your kicks as your flexibility improves, but always prioritize control and stability over distance.

✗ MISTAKES TO AVOID

- **Improper Feet Placement:** Avoid positioning your feet too low on the wall, as this can compromise stability and reduce mobility for the kick.

- **Overextending the Kick:** Focus on controlled leg movements rather than long kicks to avoid strain and losing balance.

- **Bending your knee:** While your leg starts bent, make sure it ends in a straight position when raised. This is essential for maintaining proper form, enhancing leg flexibility, and maximizing the exercise's effectiveness.

WALL SIT KICKS

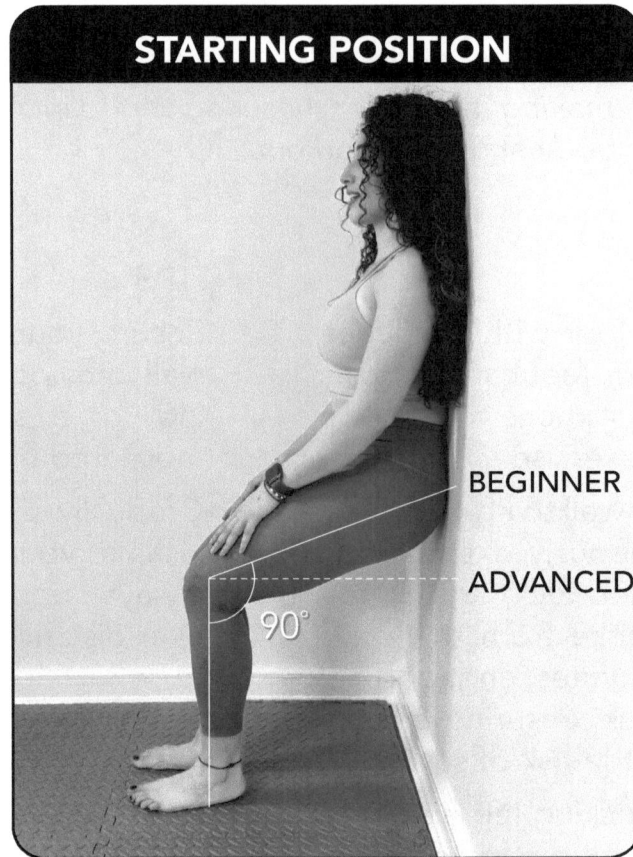

STARTING POSITION

BEGINNER

ADVANCED

90°

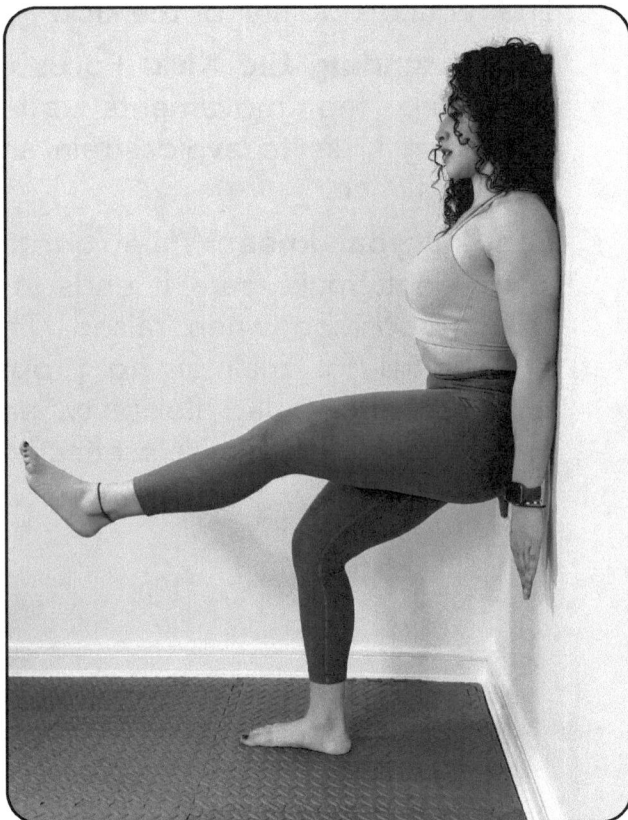

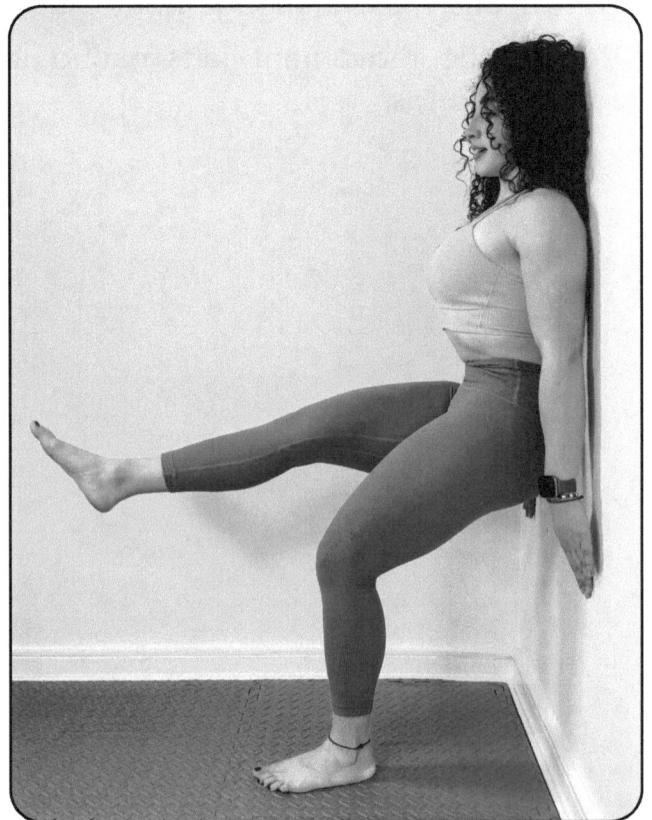

The Wall Sit Kicks exercise intensifies the traditional wall sit by adding a dynamic leg movement, significantly challenging the quadriceps and enhancing balance. This variation not only targets the thigh muscles but also engages the core, promoting stability and endurance. By extending each leg alternately while maintaining the wall sit position, this exercise isolates and activates the thigh muscles intensely while also engaging the core for better stability and posture.

INSTRUCTIONS

1. Start by standing with your back to the wall. Slide down into a seated position.

2. Engage your core and press your back and shoulders firmly against the wall.

3. Carefully extend one leg out in front of you, keeping it straight, while the other leg remains bent, supporting your body. Ensure your raised leg is parallel to the ground.

4. Hold the extension briefly, then slowly lower your leg back to the starting position.

5. Repeat the movement with the other leg, alternating between legs for each repetition.

6. Aim to repeat the kicks for 30 seconds, maintaining the wall sit posture throughout the exercise.

✓ TIPS

- Position your arms out to the sides against the wall, which will help maintain balance and provide additional support throughout the exercise.

- Beginners may start with a higher wall sit position. Gradually work your way down to a lower position where your knees are bent at a 90-degree angle, increasing the exercise's intensity over time.

- Aim to bring your raised leg parallel to the floor to maximize the exercise's benefits.

✗ MISTAKES TO AVOID

- **Avoid Arching:** Keep your lower back and shoulders pressed against the wall consistently to prevent any strain and uphold the correct posture throughout the exercise.

- **Avoid Momentum and Dropping:** Execute each leg extension with careful control and precision, ensuring you do not rely on momentum. Gradually raise and lower your leg, maintaining control throughout the entire movement to prevent any abrupt dropping.

- **Uneven Shoulders:** Watch that your shoulders don't droop or become uneven during the exercise. Proper alignment is crucial for a balanced workout.

WALL PLANK UPS

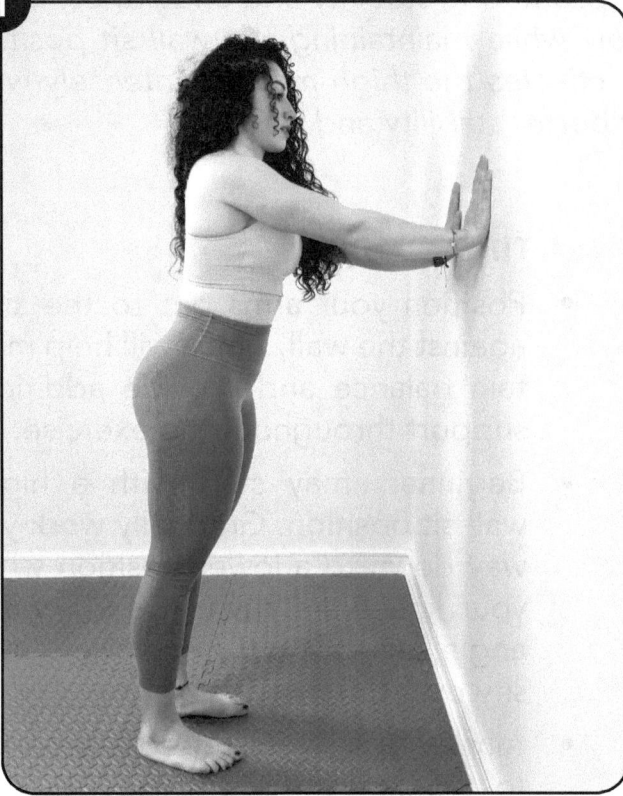

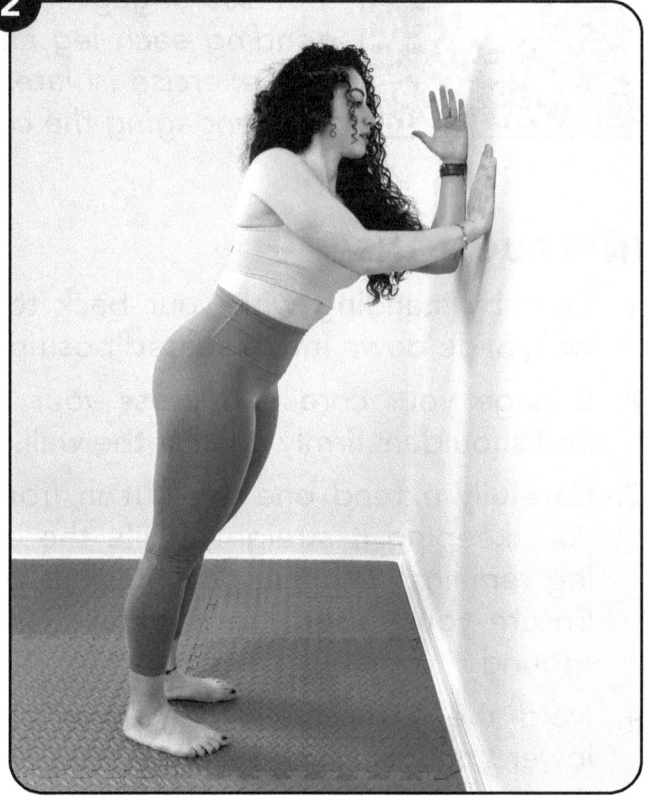

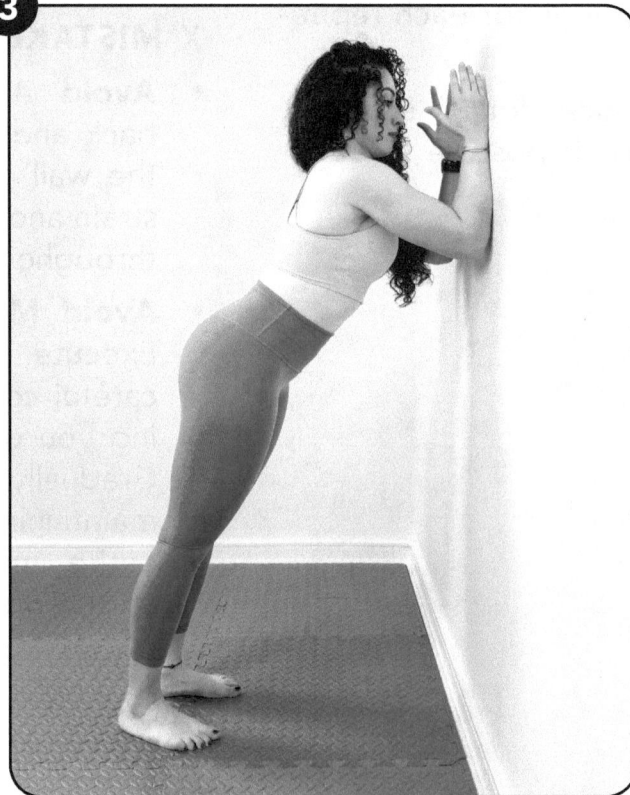

Wall Plank Ups is a variation of the traditional plank exercise, performed with palms on the wall. This exercise combines the core-engaging benefits of a plank with dynamic movement, transitioning between a high and low plank position using the wall for support. It targets the core, shoulders, chest, and triceps, enhancing upper body strength, stability, and endurance. Suitable for a range of fitness levels, Wall Plank Ups offers a unique challenge to the classic floor-based plank ups.

INSTRUCTIONS

1. Stand facing the wall, approximately an arm's length away. Place your palms on the wall at shoulder height, assuming a standing plank position with your body in a straight line from head to heels.

2. Bend one elbow to bring your forearm to the wall.

3. Bend the other elbow, transitioning into a low plank with both forearms resting on the wall.

   Press one hand back up to the starting position, followed by the other, returning to the high plank with palms on the wall.

   Continue alternating between the high and low plank positions, maintaining a strong core and straight body line throughout the exercise.

   Perform the exercise for a set duration or number of repetitions, focusing on controlled and stable transitions.

✓ TIPS

- Keep your core engaged at all times to support your lower back and maintain proper alignment.

- Ensure smooth and controlled transitions between high and low plank positions to maximize muscle engagement and stability.

- Adjust your distance from the wall to control intensity: stepping closer reduces difficulty, while moving further away increases the challenge.

✗ MISTAKES TO AVOID

- **Sagging Hips:** Avoid letting your hips sag or pike up, as this can compromise the effectiveness of the plank and strain your lower back.

- **Rushing Transitions:** Do not rush the movement between high and low planks. Controlled, deliberate movements ensure better muscle activation and prevent loss of form.

- **Misaligning Shoulders:** Keep your shoulders directly over your wrists in the high plank and your elbows in the low plank to ensure proper form.

SHOULDER TAPS

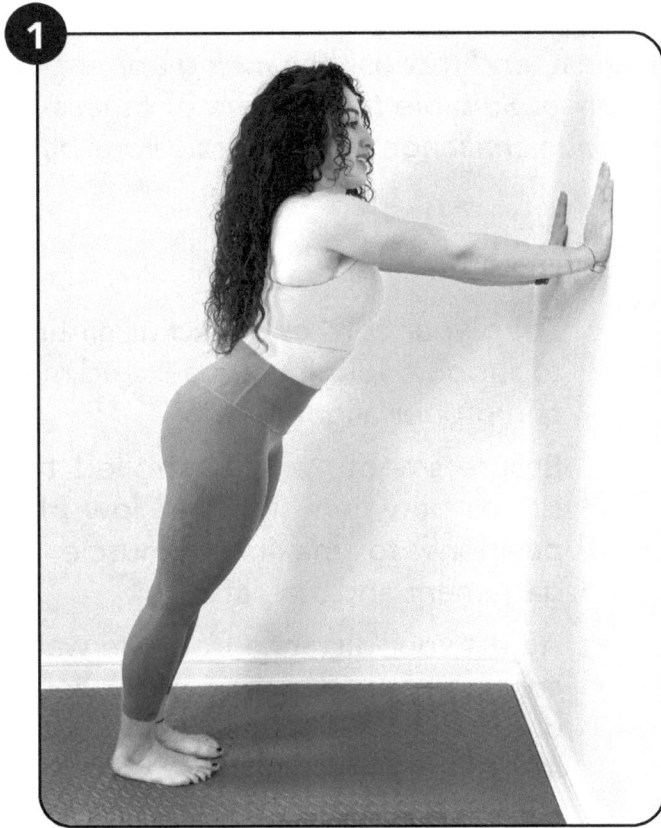

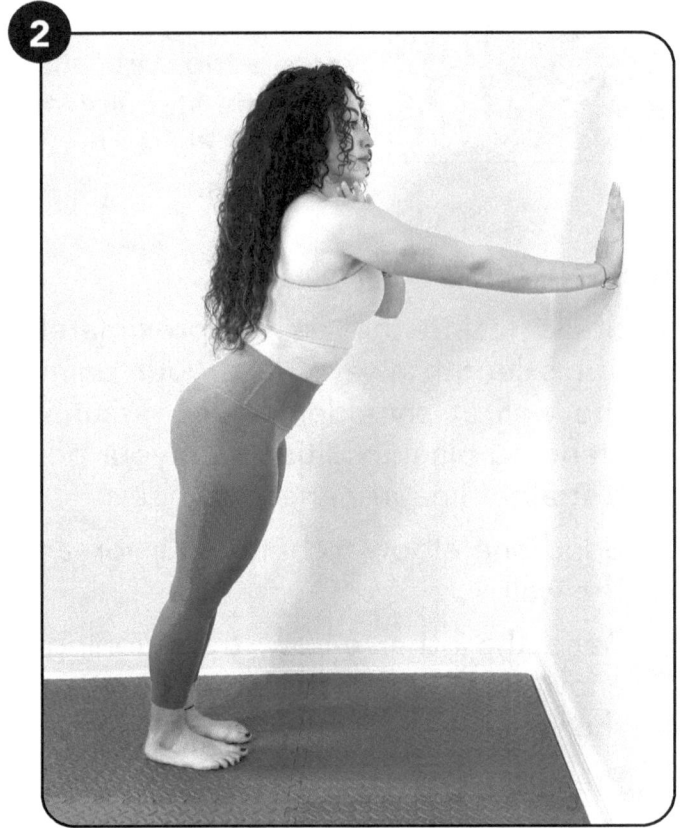

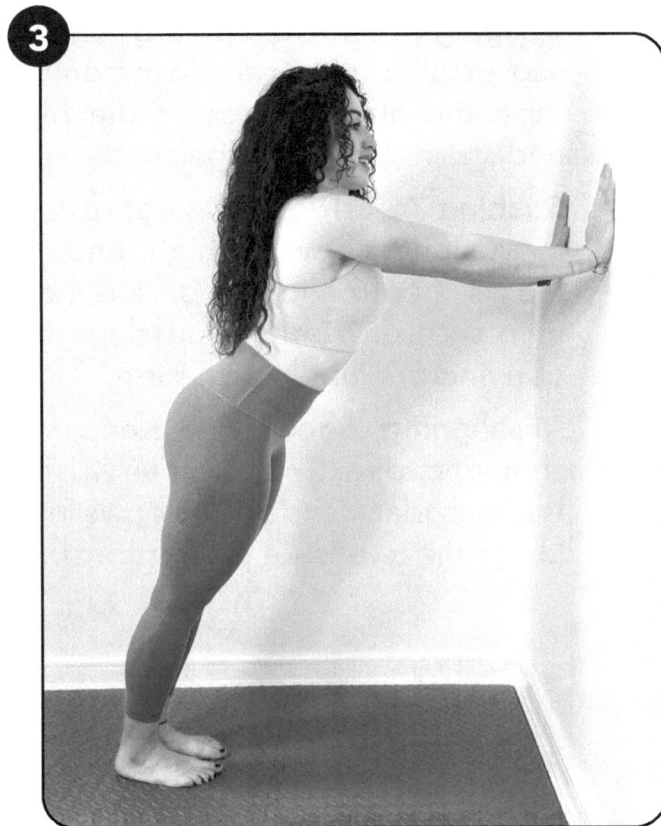

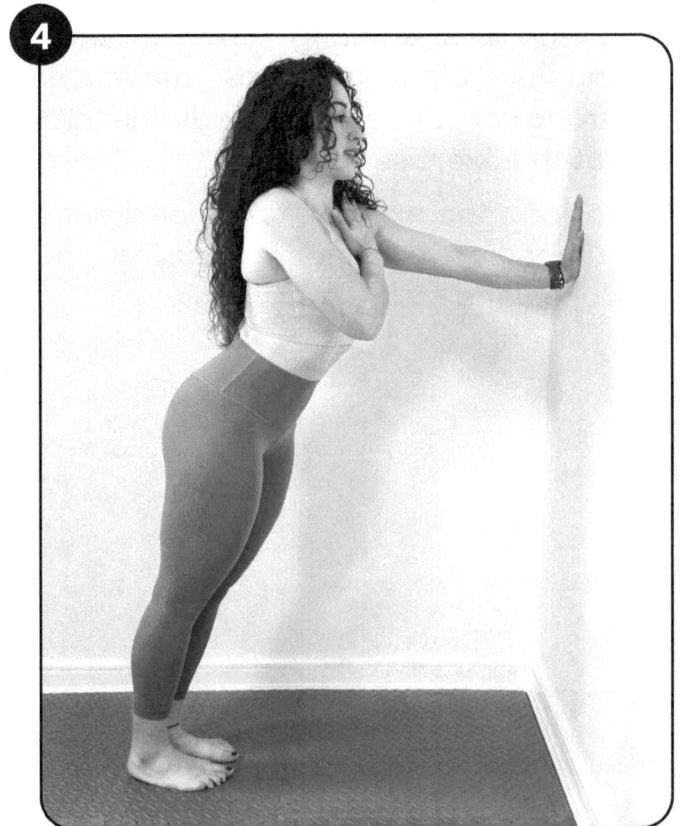

Shoulder Taps are a dynamic variation of the traditional plank exercise, performed with palms against the wall. This exercise engages the core, shoulders, and arms by adding the movement of tapping the opposite shoulder with each hand. The wall support decreases the intensity compared to floor-based shoulder taps, making it accessible for beginners or those focusing on upper body stability and coordination.

INSTRUCTIONS

1. Stand facing the wall, slightly more than an arm's length away. Place your palms on the wall at shoulder height, keeping your feet shoulder-width apart to assume a standing plank position.

2. Shift your weight slightly to the right and lift your left hand off the wall to tap your right shoulder, aiming to keep your hips and shoulders as stable as possible.

3. Return your left hand to the wall, reverting to the starting position.

4. Repeat the motion by lifting your right hand to tap your left shoulder, making sure to keep your core engaged and strong throughout the movement.

   Continue alternating shoulder taps, focusing on controlled movements and stability. Perform the exercise for a set duration or number of repetitions.

✓ TIPS

- Keep your body in a straight line from head to heels, engaging your core to prevent the hips from swaying.

- Perform the taps slowly and deliberately to maintain balance and maximize muscle engagement.

- To increase the challenge, move your feet closer together to decrease stability and increase the demand on your core.

✗ MISTAKES TO AVOID

- **Rotating the Hips:** Avoid letting your hips rotate or lift as you perform the taps. Aim to keep your lower body stable to engage the core effectively.

- **Losing Form:** Ensure not to sag your lower back or pike your hips up. Keep your body aligned and steady

- **Rushing the Movement:** Resist the temptation to speed through the taps. Slow, controlled taps ensure better stability and muscle activation.

FLEX UP TO TOES

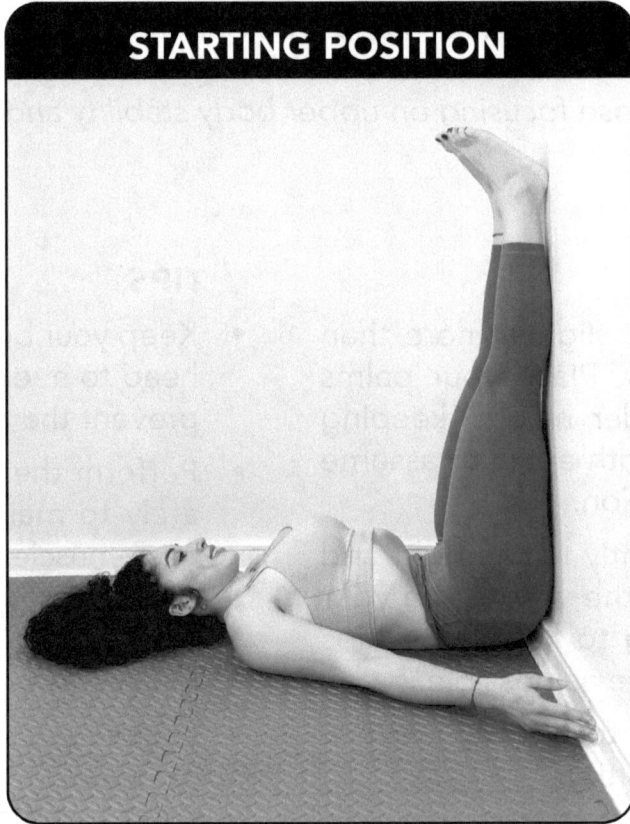

STARTING POSITION

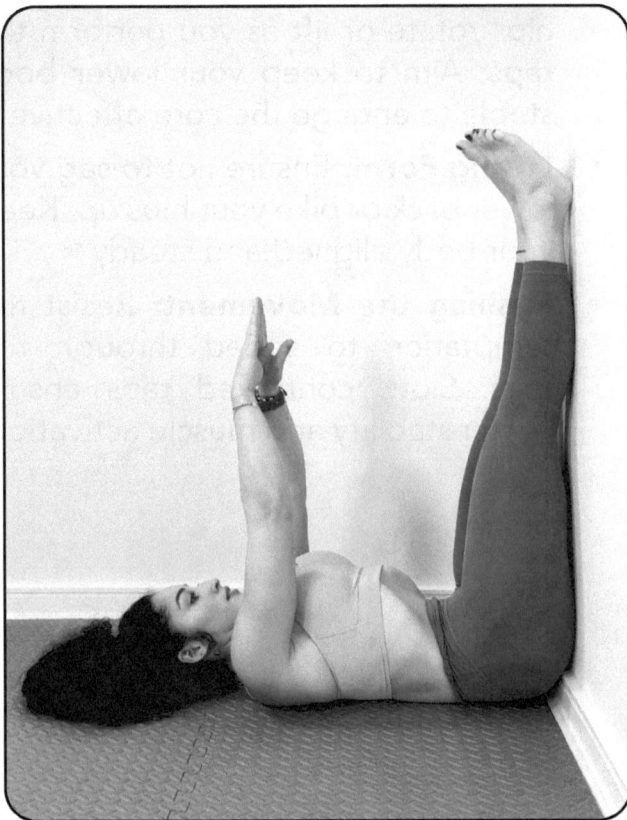

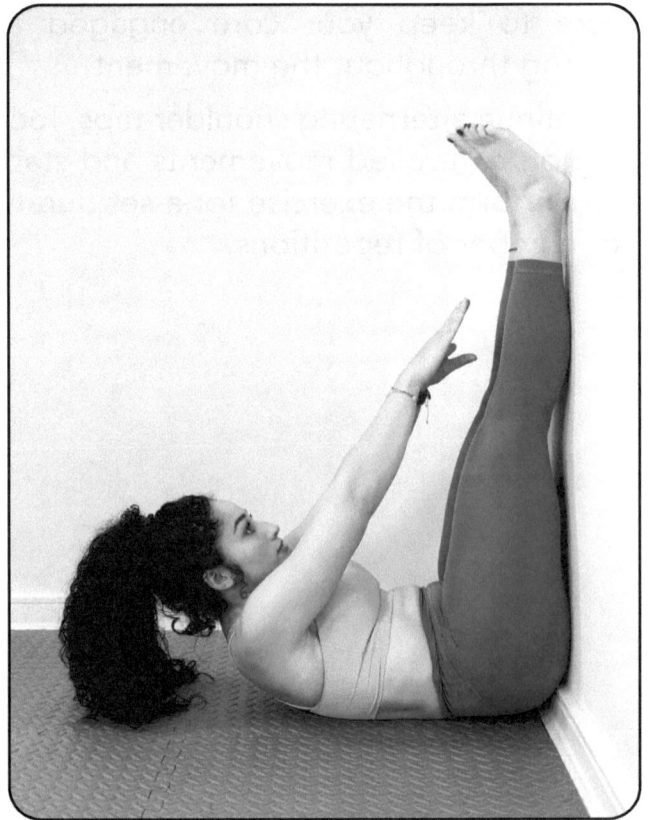

Wall Flex Up to Toes is a core-strengthening exercise that combines the stability of a wall-supported leg position with the dynamic movement of a crunch. Starting with the back on the floor and legs fully supported by the wall, this exercise targets the abdominal muscles by flexing upwards to reach the toes with the hands. The sustained flex-up position enhances muscle engagement and endurance, making it an effective workout for improving core strength and flexibility.

INSTRUCTIONS

1. Lie on your back on the floor, placing your legs straight up against the wall. Make sure your entire legs, from glutes to feet, are in full contact with the wall.

2. Raise your arms towards the ceiling, keeping them parallel to your legs and the wall, with your fingers pointing upwards.

3. Engage your abdominal muscles and slowly lift your upper body off the floor, reaching towards your toes with your hands. Maintain this flexed position up to three seconds to maximize core engagement.

4. Gently lower your upper body back to the floor, maintaining control and keeping your arms raised.

5. Continue with the flex-ups, focusing on controlled, precise movements. Perform the exercise for a predetermined number of repetitions or a specific duration, ensuring consistent form and engagement.

✓ TIPS

- Breathe out as you flex up and breathe in as you return to the starting position to maintain a rhythmic breathing pattern.

- For correct posture during exercises, direct your gaze towards your feet in both positions: while lying down on the floor and while flexing up. This approach ensures a neutral neck alignment and reduces stress on your neck.

- To ensure your legs are fully extended along the wall, begin by sitting as close to it as possible, then place your feet against the wall. Use your arms to push your body closer until your glutes are also touching the wall, then carefully lie down on the floor.

✗ MISTAKES TO AVOID

- **Losing Leg Position:** Ensure your legs remain fully supported by the wall throughout the exercise to maintain proper form and stability.

- **Jerking Movements:** Avoid using momentum to lift your upper body. Focus on controlled, smooth movements to effectively engage the core.

- **Straining the Neck:** Avoid pulling your neck forward or excessively tucking your chin during the flex-up. Maintain a neutral neck position, directing your gaze towards your feet to help guide and ensure proper posture.

TWIST TO KNEE

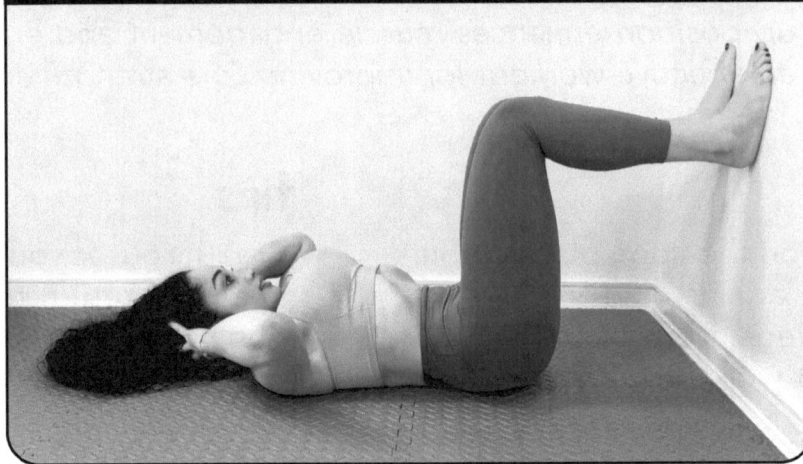
STARTING POSITION

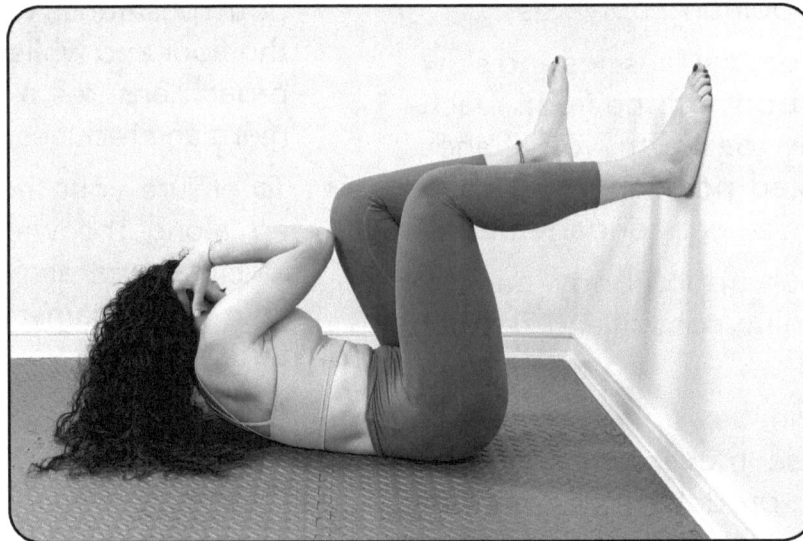

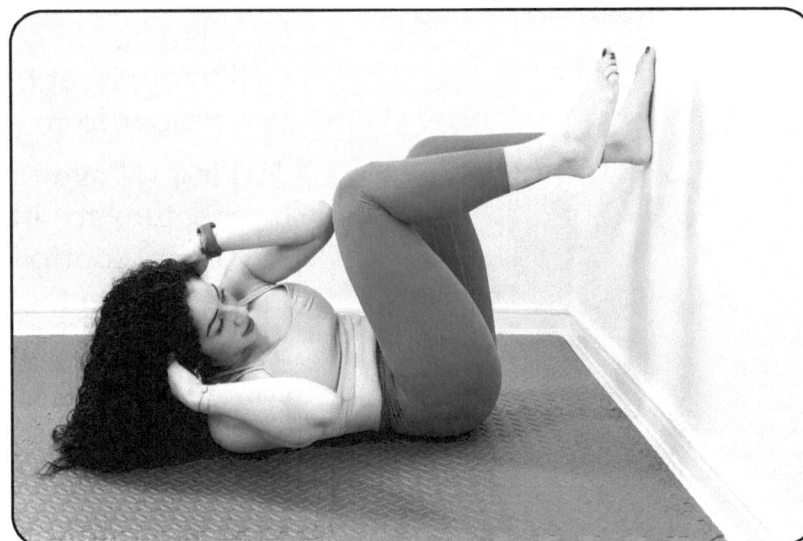

The Twist to Knee on the wall is a core exercise that adapts the classic bicycle crunch movement to a wall-supported format. With feet placed against the wall and legs bent at a 90-degree angle, this exercise involves twisting movements targeting the obliques and engaging the entire abdominal region. It's an effective workout for enhancing core strength, flexibility, and coordination, with the added stability of the wall aiding in maintaining proper form.

INSTRUCTIONS

1. Lie on your back on the floor with your feet flat against the wall, knees bent at a 90-degree angle. Place your hands behind your head for support.

2. Engage your core and slightly lift one shoulder off the floor, twisting your torso. Simultaneously, bring the opposite knee closer to your chest, keeping the other foot flat on the wall. Aim to touch the lifted knee with the opposite elbow.

3. Gently lower your foot back to the wall and your shoulder to the floor. Repeat the twist on the other side, lifting the other leg.

4. Continue alternating legs and twisting your upper body from side to side in a controlled bicycle motion.

5. Aim for a set number of repetitions or a specific duration, focusing on smooth, controlled movements and consistent core engagement.

✓ TIPS

- Keep your elbows wide and avoid pulling on your neck with your hands to ensure proper form and prevent strain.

- Breathe out as you twist to each side and inhale as you return to the center to maintain a rhythmic breathing pattern.

- Hold the flex-up position for a few seconds to further engage your core throughout the exercise.

- To add more challenge, begin with your legs straight against the wall instead of bent. Maintain the same distance from the wall as if your knees were bent. This position increases engagement in the lower body, particularly in the leg muscles and glutes.

✗ MISTAKES TO AVOID

- **Don't Overstretch:** Avoid overstretching your torso while twisting. It's fine if your knee and elbow don't touch; flexibility will improve with practice.

- **Jerky Movements:** Avoid rapid, uncontrolled twists, as this can reduce the effectiveness of the exercise and increase the risk of injury.

- **Straining the Neck:** Ensure your neck remains relaxed, with the twist coming from your core rather than pulling with your hands.

FLEX UP ALTERNATE ARMS

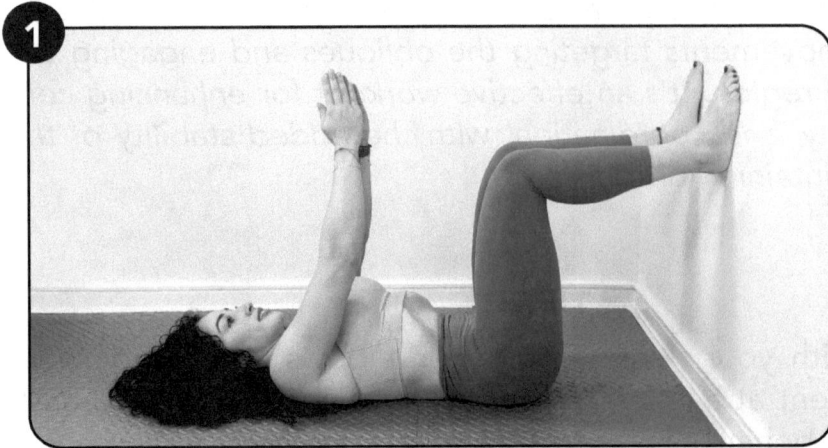

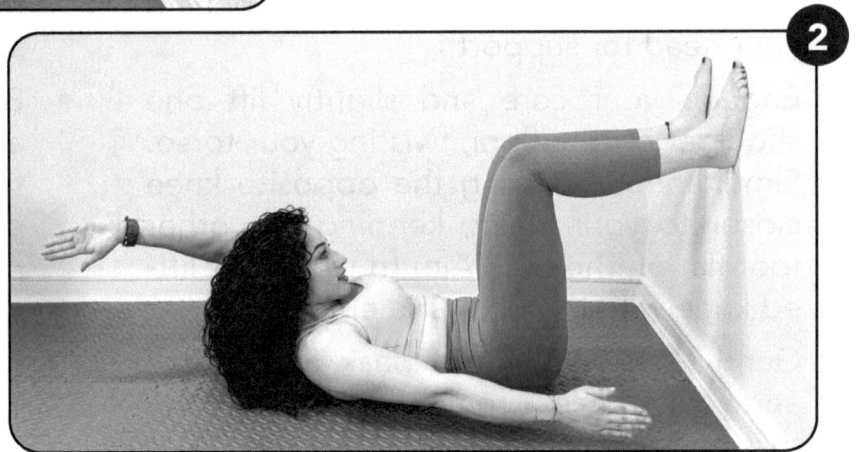

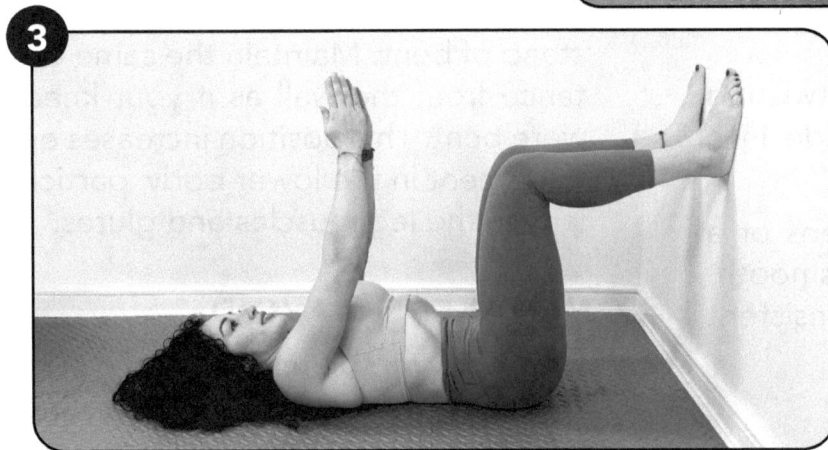

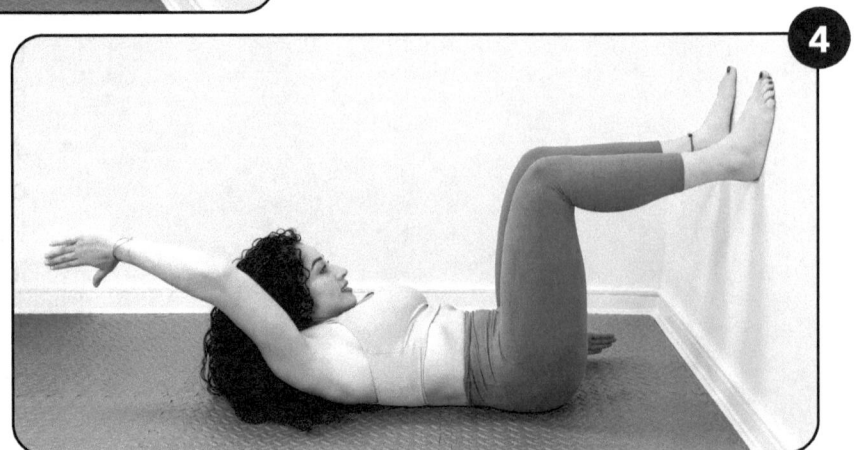

The Flex Up Alternate Arms is a core-strengthening exercise that incorporates an upper body movement to enhance the challenge. This exercise targets the abdominal muscles while engaging the shoulders and arms through alternating arm movements during the flex-up motion. It's ideal for improving core stability, upper body strength, and coordination.

INSTRUCTIONS

1. Lie on your back on the floor with your feet flat against the wall, knees bent at a 90-degree angle. Extend your arms towards the ceiling with palms facing each other, head and back resting on the floor.

2. Engage your core and perform a flex-up, simultaneously lowering one arm down to your side and extending the other arm overhead.

3. Slowly lower back down to the starting position, bringing both arms back up towards the ceiling.

4. Repeat the flex-up motion, this time switching the positions of your arms (the arm that was overhead moves down to your side, and the arm that was at your side extends overhead).

   Alternate the arm positions with each flex-up, focusing on controlled movements and core engagement. Perform the exercise for a set number of repetitions or duration.

✓ TIPS

- Keep your chin slightly tucked to maintain a neutral neck position and avoid straining.

- Ensure a smooth transition between arms for better coordination and focus on core engagement.

- Breathe out as you flex up and breathe in as you return to the starting position to maintain a steady breathing rhythm.

✗ MISTAKES TO AVOID

- **Overextending Arms:** Be cautious not to overstretch, especially the arm extending overhead, as this may cause discomfort or injuries. The goal isn't to touch the floor but to keep your core and upper body engaged. Ensure you maintain a controlled range of motion.

- **Arching the Back:** Keep your lower back pressed against the floor to prevent arching and ensure the core is effectively engaged.

- **Jerky Movements:** Avoid rapid or uncontrolled movements; each flex-up and arm movement should be smooth and deliberate.

- **Losing Focus on the Core:** Ensure the primary focus remains on engaging the abdominal muscles throughout the exercise, rather than the arm movements dominating the action.

AB CRUNCH + MARCH

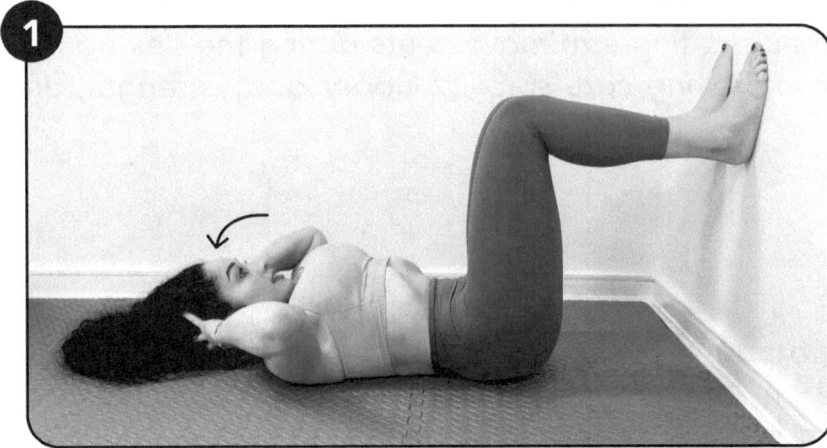

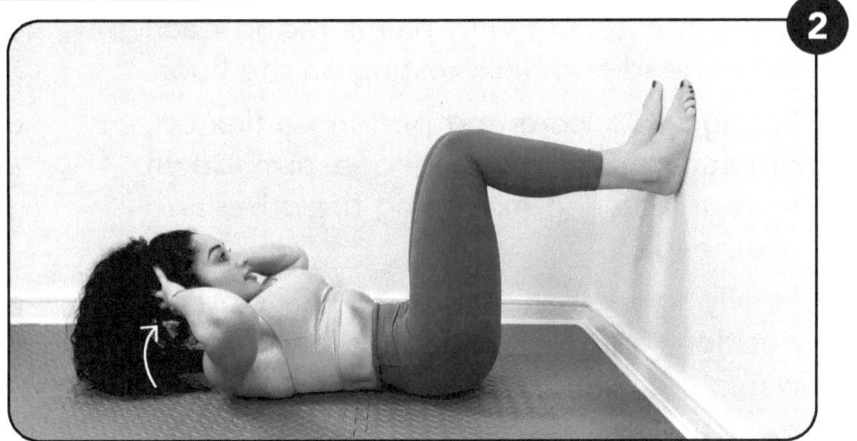

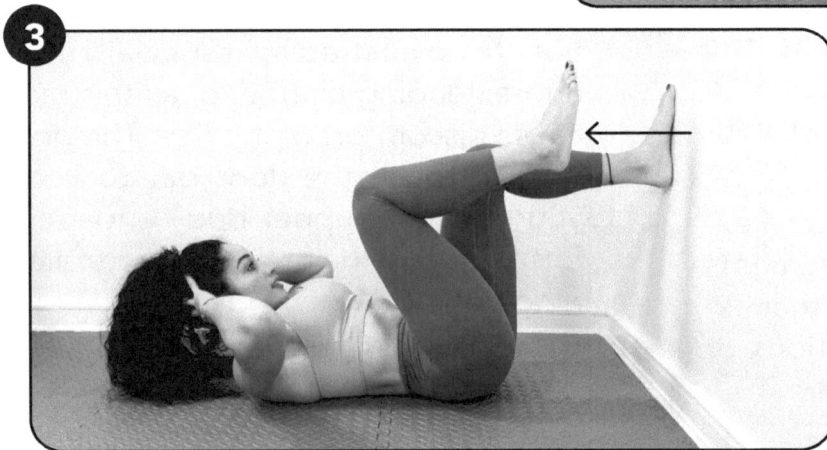

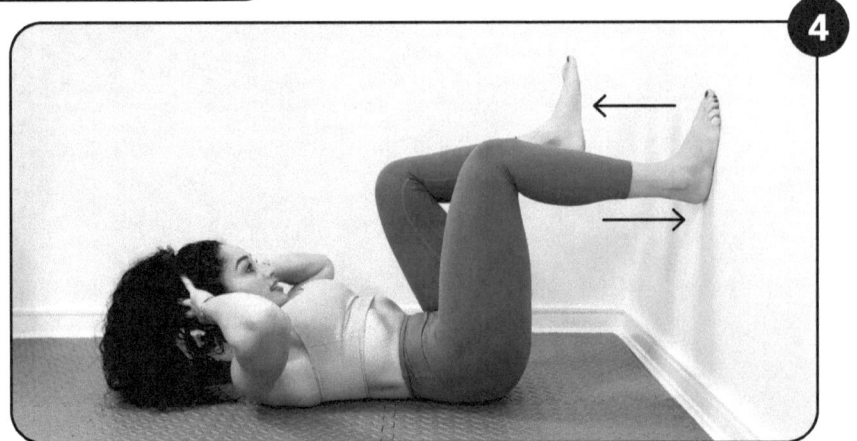

The Ab Crunch Plus March on the wall is a compound exercise that combines traditional abdominal crunches with a marching motion, all while utilizing the wall for leg support. This exercise engages the core, hip flexors, and glutes, enhancing core strength, lower body endurance, and coordination. It's particularly effective for targeting multiple muscle groups simultaneously, making it a comprehensive workout for the abdominals and legs.

INSTRUCTIONS

1. Lie on your back on the floor with your legs raised and feet flat against the wall, knees bent at a 90-degree angle. Place your hands lightly behind your head or crossed over your chest, with your head and back resting on the floor.

2. Engage your core and lift your upper body off the floor into a crunch, ensuring your lower back remains pressed down.

3. While holding the crunch position, lift one foot off the wall, drawing the knee closer to your chest.

4. Gently return the foot to the wall and stabilize your position before lifting the other foot.

   After returning the second foot to the wall, release the crunch by lowering your head and shoulders to the floor.

   Perform the exercise for a set number of repetitions or duration.

✓ TIPS

• Maintain a steady pace, synchronizing the crunch with the marching motion to enhance coordination and muscle activation.

• Inhale as you lower down and exhale as you crunch up and march, keeping your breaths synchronized with your movements for better stability and effectiveness.

• Make sure your feet are stable on the wall before changing position.

✗ MISTAKES TO AVOID

• **Pulling on the Neck:** Ensure your hands are only lightly supporting your head to avoid straining the neck during crunches.

• **Losing Wall Contact:** Keep one foot in constant contact with the wall to ensure stability and proper form during the marching motion.

• **Rushing the Movements:** Avoid fast, jerky movements. Each crunch and march should be performed with intention and control to prevent momentum from reducing the exercise's effectiveness.

TIPS UP TO HEEL

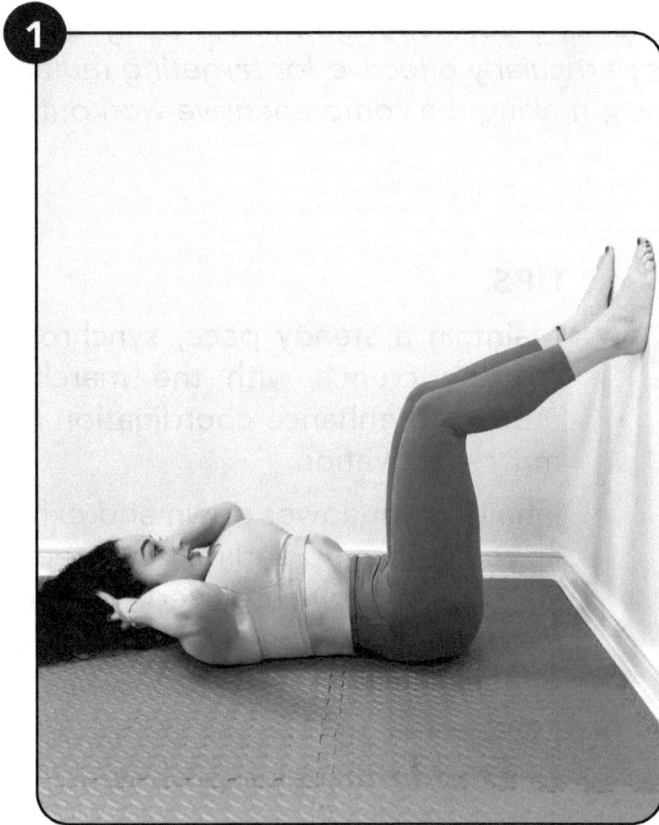

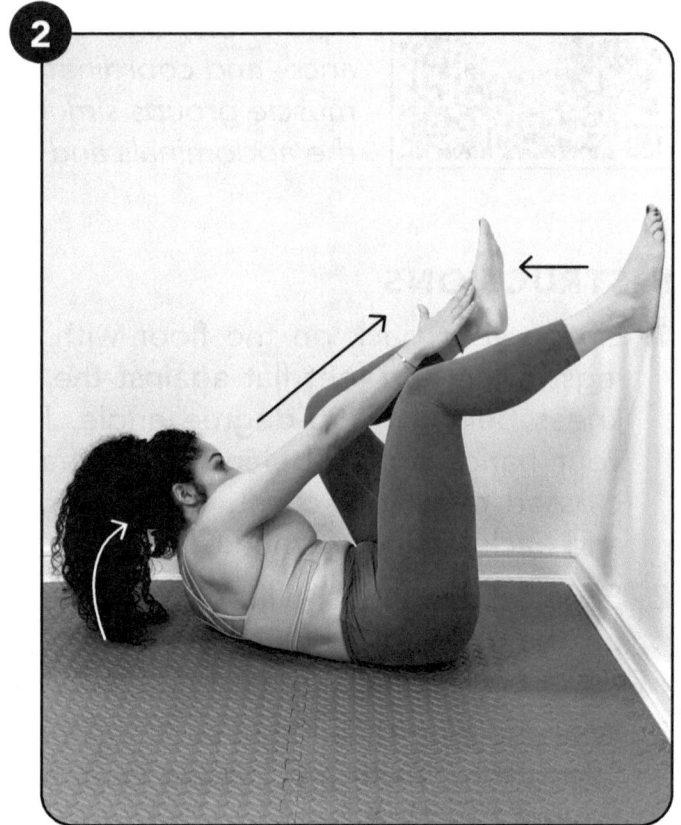

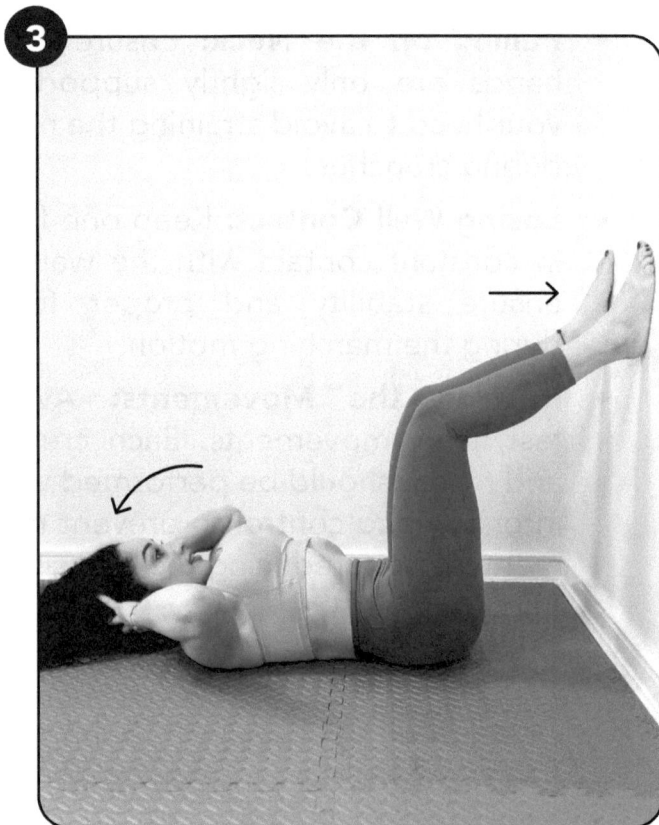

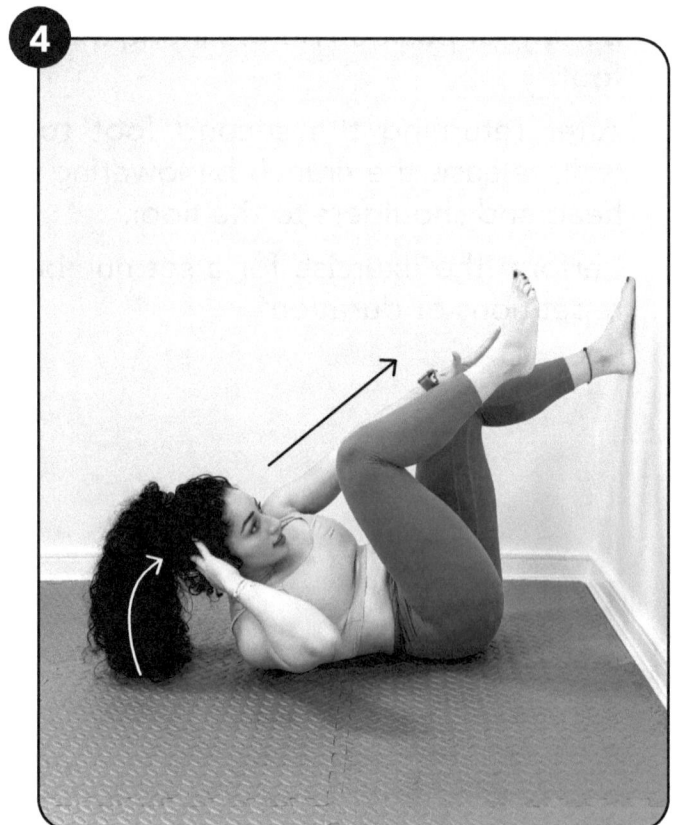

Tips Up to Heel is a dynamic core exercise that incorporates elements of the traditional bicycle exercise with a unique twist. Performed with feet against the wall, this exercise targets the abdominal muscles, obliques, and improves coordination. This exercise not only targets the core and oblique muscles but also introduces an element of stability and precision through the use of the wall. As participants strive to touch their heel with the opposite hand, they benefit from improved muscular endurance and flexibility.

INSTRUCTIONS

1. Lie on your back on the floor, with your feet flat against the wall and knees slightly bent. Place your hands behind your head for support, ensuring your elbows are kept wide apart.

2. Engage your core and twist your torso, lifting one leg off the wall. Simultaneously, reach with the opposite hand to touch the heel of the lifted leg.

3. With control, return to the starting position by lowering your shoulders to the floor and bringing the lifted leg back to the wall.

4. Repeat the motion on the other side, lifting the other leg while aiming to touch its heel with the opposite hand while twisting your torso.

   Continue the exercise for a set number of repetitions or for a specific duration. Ensure you return to the starting position after each twist before switching sides.

✓ TIPS

- Coordinate your breath with your movements—inhale as you return to the starting position and exhale during the twist and leg lift to maintain a steady rhythm.

- Emphasize slow, controlled movements rather than speed to maximize engagement and effectiveness of the exercise.

- It's more beneficial to perform the exercise with correct form than to reach the heel at the cost of twisting improperly.

✗ MISTAKES TO AVOID

- **Don't Lower Your Legs Too Down:** Make small movements with your legs, focusing more on engaging your core rather than making large, sweeping motions.

- **Don't Overstretch:** Don't worry if you cannot make contact with your feet or heel initially. Just touch the leg wherever you can comfortably reach. Flexibility will improve with practice.

- **Don't Pull with Your Hands and Neck:** Instead of using your hands to pull your neck or forcing the movement, engage your core to perform the twists and lifts. This ensures the movement is driven by your core muscles, not your neck or arms.

WALL CHILD TO PLANK

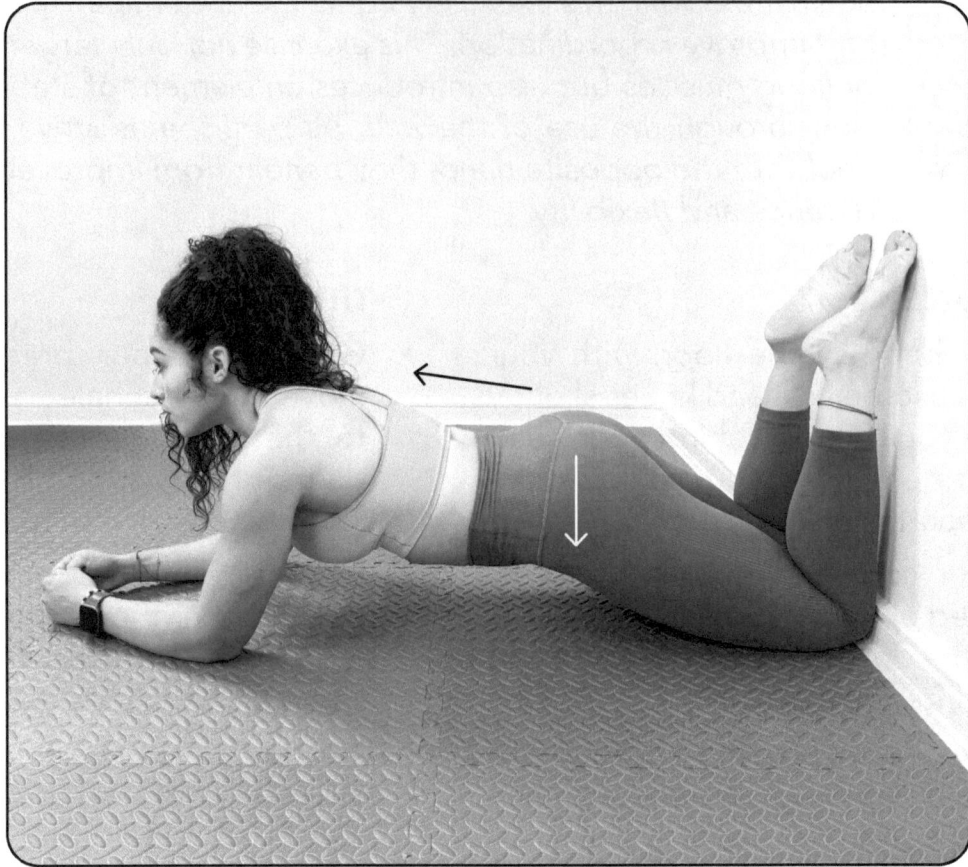

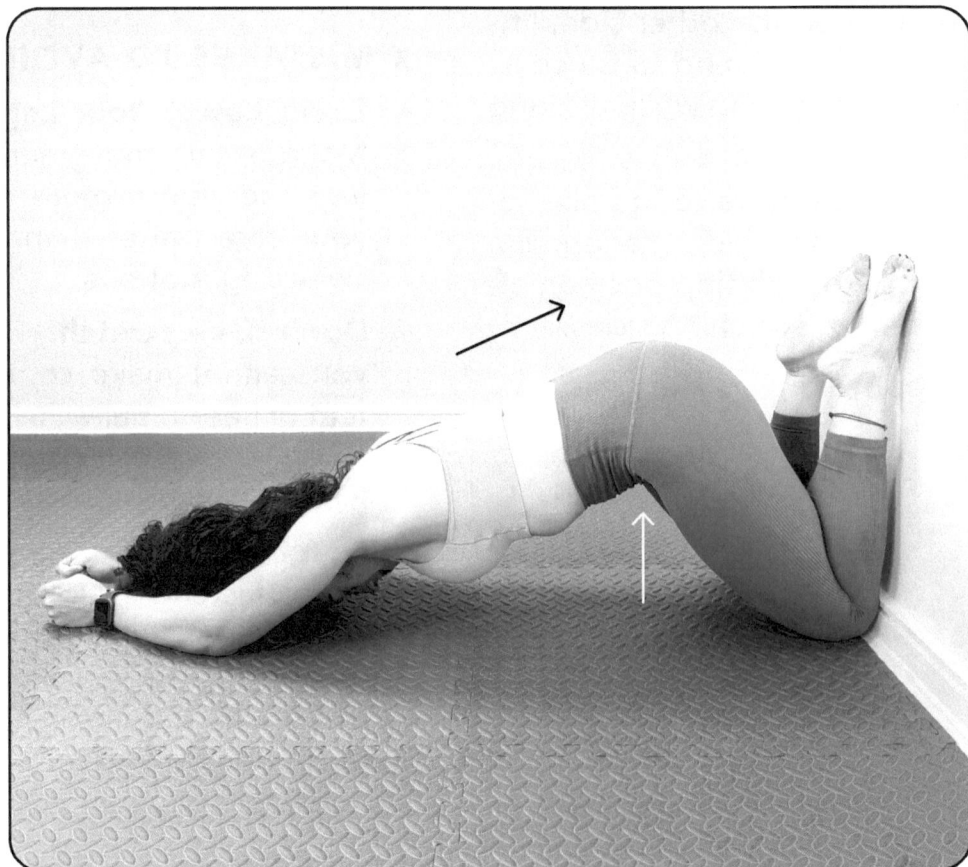

The Wall Child to Plank exercise is a bodyweight movement that blends the stability and core engagement of a plank with the hip and lower back stretch of the child's pose, using the wall for added resistance and form refinement. This exercise enhances core strength, promotes spinal alignment, and increases flexibility in the legs, making it a versatile addition to any fitness routine.

INSTRUCTIONS

1. Lie prone on the mat, facing down, with your knees at the base of the wall and shins pressed against it. Position your arms on the mat with elbows directly your shoulders.

2. Activate your core muscles to lift your chest and hips off the mat. Your body should form a straight line from head to knees, similar to a plank position.

3. While keeping your forearms and elbows stationary, engage your glutes to lift and push them back towards your feet, creating a modified child's pose with your shins against the wall. Your arms should extend almost straight, providing a gentle back stretch.

4. Carefully lower your hips back down, transitioning into the plank position again. Maintain constant pressure against the wall with your shins and knees.

5. Continue the movement between these two positions for the desired number of repetitions or time duration.

✓ TIP

- Focus on controlled breathing, inhaling during the transition to the child's pose and exhaling as you return to the plank.

✗ MISTAKES TO AVOID

- **Avoid disengaging your core:** Ensure constant engagement of your core to prevent your hips and abdomen from touching the mat. Continuous core activation is crucial to stabilize your body and enhance the effectiveness of the transition between poses.

- **Forearm Instability:** Maintain the position of your forearms without allowing them to slide. Using a yoga mat or a non-slip surface can help keep your forearms anchored.

WALL-SUPPORTED KNEE RAISE

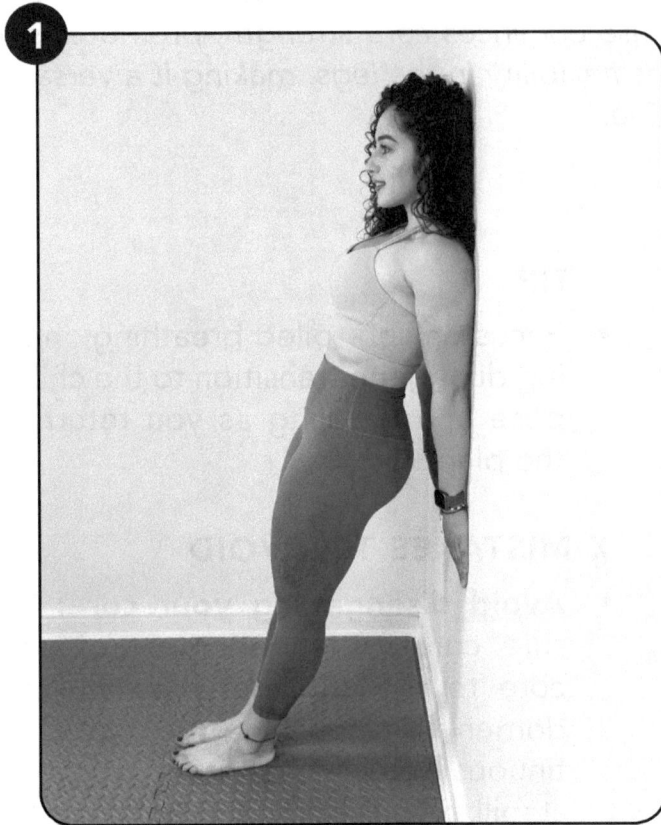

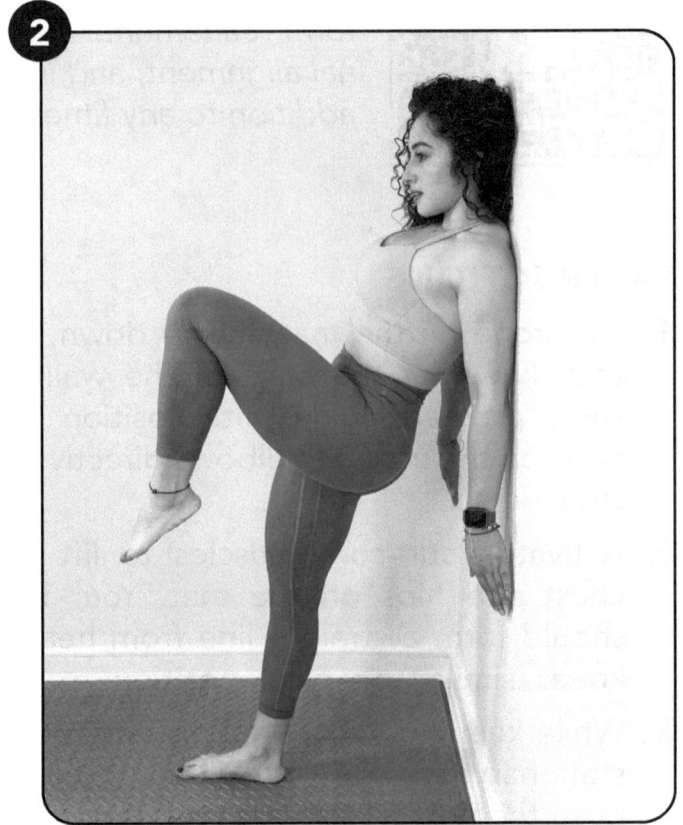

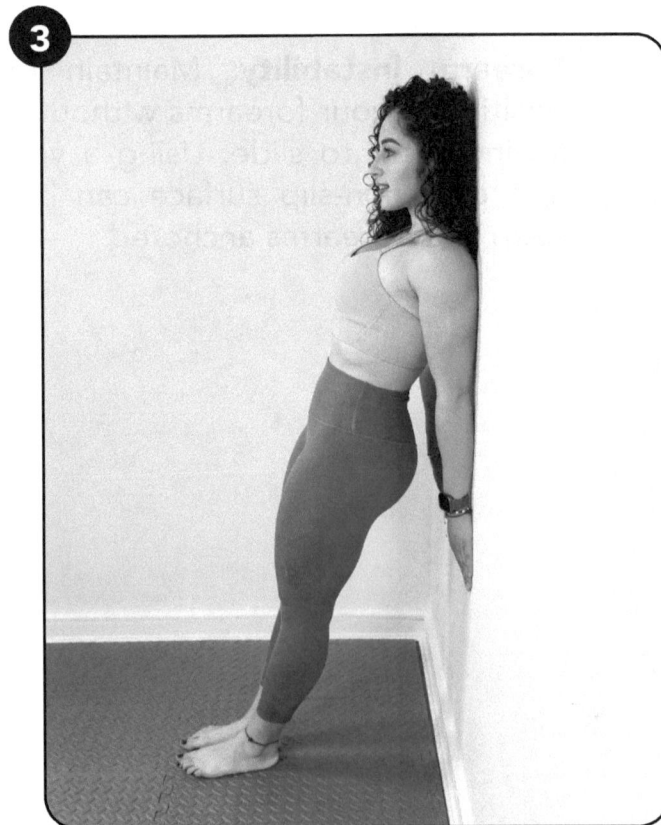

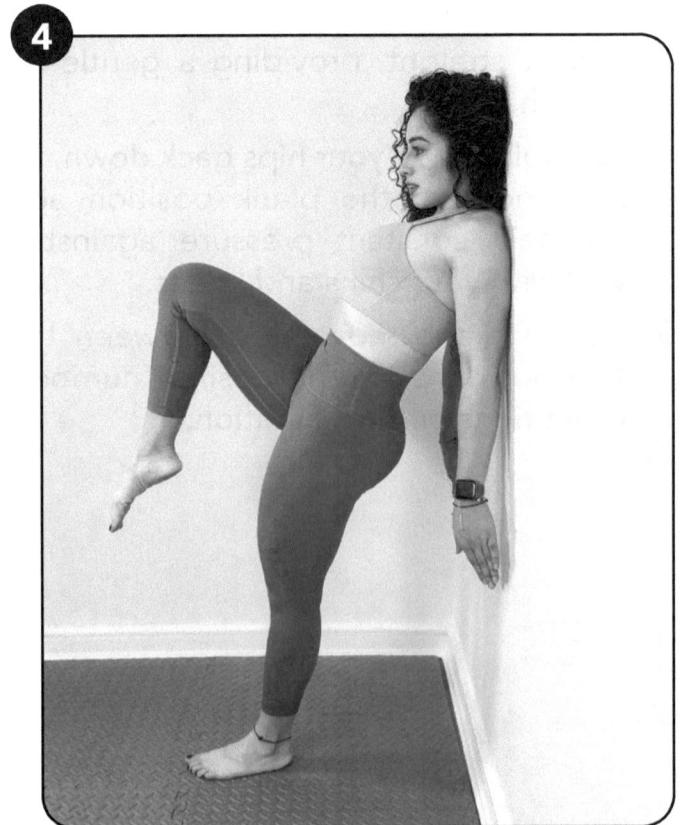

The Wall-Supported Knee Raise is a targeted exercise that strengthens the lower abdominal muscles and hip flexors. By performing this movement against the wall, you gain additional stability, allowing for more focused muscle engagement. It's particularly beneficial for enhancing core stability and improving hip mobility.

INSTRUCTIONS

1. Start by leaning your upper back against the wall. Step your feet forward about two feet from the wall, keeping them together. Place your hands against the wall for added support.

2. Slowly lift one knee toward your chest without arching your lower back, keeping the movement controlled and focused on engaging your lower abs.

3. Lower your knee back to the starting position in a controlled manner.

4. Repeat the movement with the other knee.

   Aim to repeat the exercise for 30 seconds, focusing on maintaining constant contact with the wall and engaging your core throughout the exercise.

✓ TIPS

- Concentrate on engaging your core muscles as you lift your knee, imagining you're trying to touch your chest with your knee without rounding your back.

- Focus on breathing steadily throughout the exercise; exhale as you lift your knee and inhale as you lower it.

- To increase the challenge, try holding the raised knee position for a few seconds before lowering.

✗ MISTAKES TO AVOID

- **Standing Too Far from the Wall:** Avoid standing too far as it might lead to an exaggerated back arch, undermining the exercise's effectiveness and risking discomfort.

- **Standing Too Close to the Wall:** Being too close to the wall reduces the intensity of lower abs engagement and affects stability. Ideal positioning is around two feet away to effectively engage muscles and sustain proper balance.

- **Compromised Stability:** Neglecting to secure your footing can lead to slips or falls. Always use a yoga mat or wear training shoes to guarantee a stable base during your exercise.

DONKEY KICK

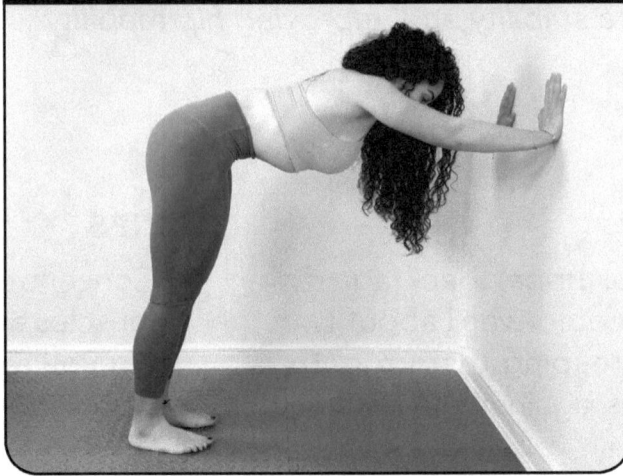

RIGHT

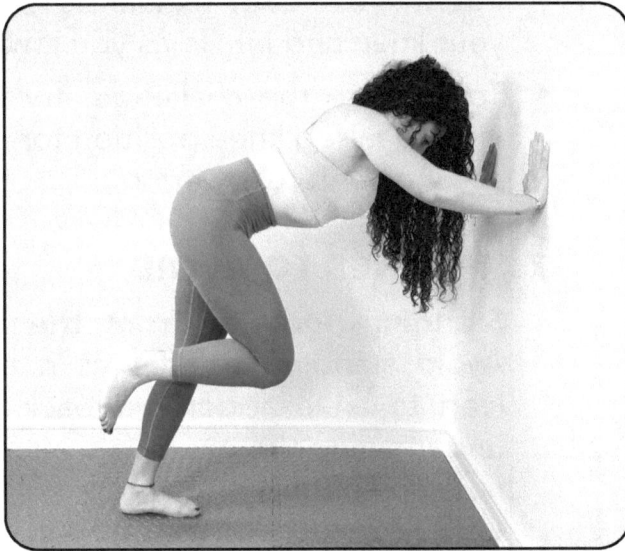

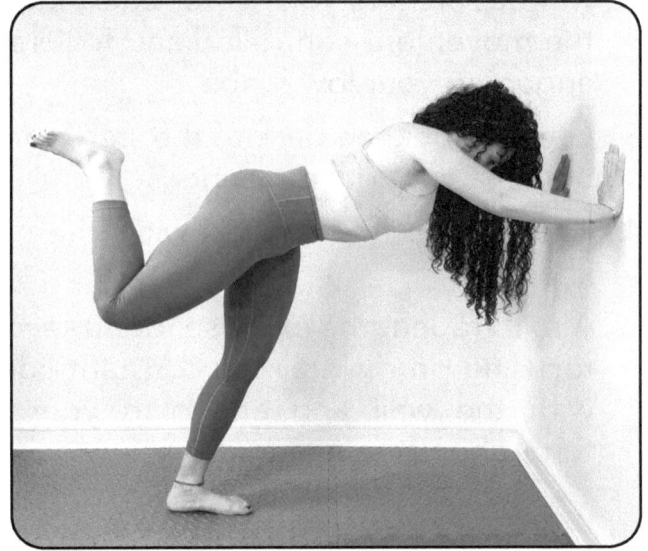

LEFT

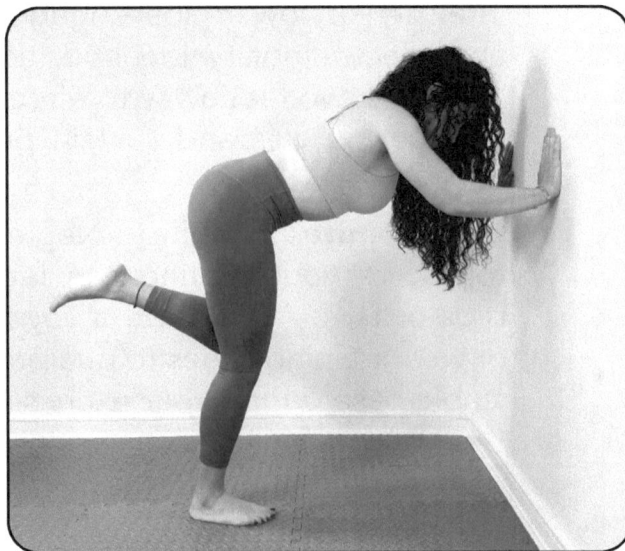

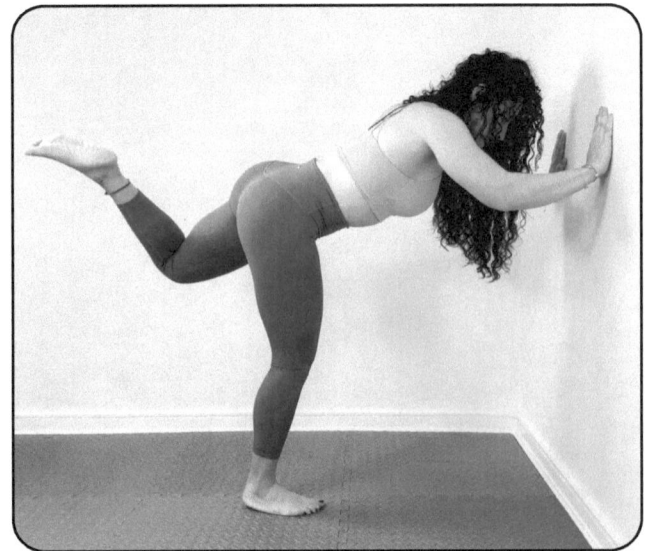

The Wall-Supported Donkey Kick targets essential lower body muscles, providing a unique approach to glute and hamstring conditioning. By utilizing the wall for support, this exercise allows for deeper muscle activation and a higher focus on technique. It's an excellent choice for anyone looking to add variety to their lower body routine and build strength in these crucial areas.

INSTRUCTIONS

1. Begin by standing an arm's length away from the wall, facing it. Place your palms against the wall at shoulder height.

2. Take a small step back and lean forward, bending at your hips until your torso is almost parallel to the floor, ensuring your arms follow the same alignment.

3. Maintain one leg straight and firmly planted on the floor for balance. With the other leg, bend the knee then lift this leg towards the ceiling. Engage your glutes to push your foot upwards, keeping your hips square to the wall. Avoid any twisting.

4. Slowly lower the lifted leg back down, maintaining the bend in the knee throughout the movement.

5. Repeat for 30 seconds before switching to the other, ensuring you maintain consistent form and engagement of your glutes throughout each repetition.

✓ TIPS

- Ensure your hands are firmly pressed against the wall throughout the exercise to maintain stability.

- Focus on squeezing your glutes as you lift your leg to maximize muscle engagement.

- For an added challenge, you can add ankle weights or resistance bands once you are comfortable with the basic movement.

✗ MISTAKES TO AVOID

- **Hip Twisting:** Avoid letting your hips twist or rotate. Keep them square to the wall to ensure proper alignment and effective muscle engagement.

- **Rushing:** Perform each repetition slowly and with control to prevent using momentum instead of muscle engagement.

WALL PUSH-UPS

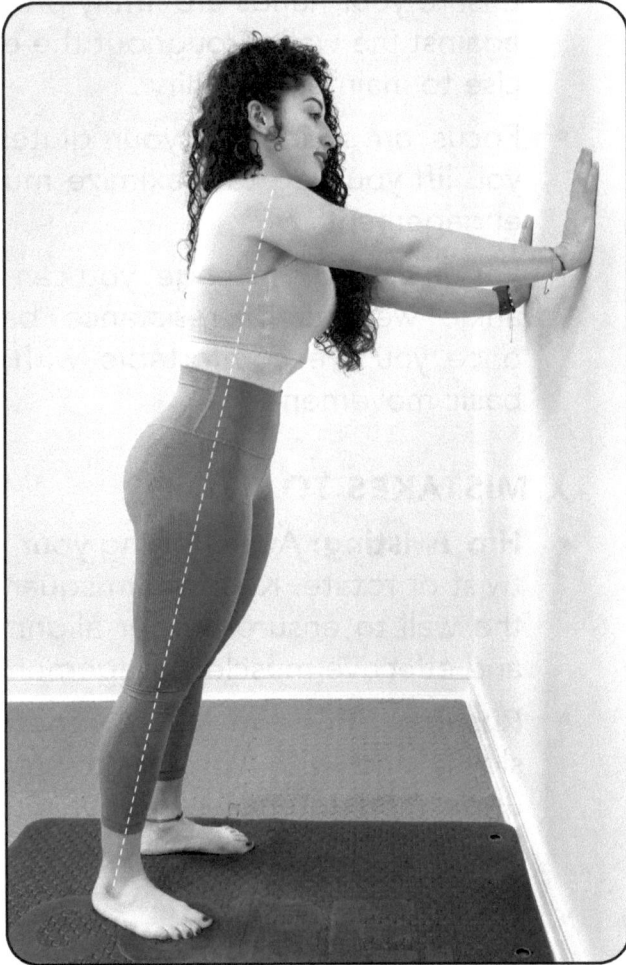
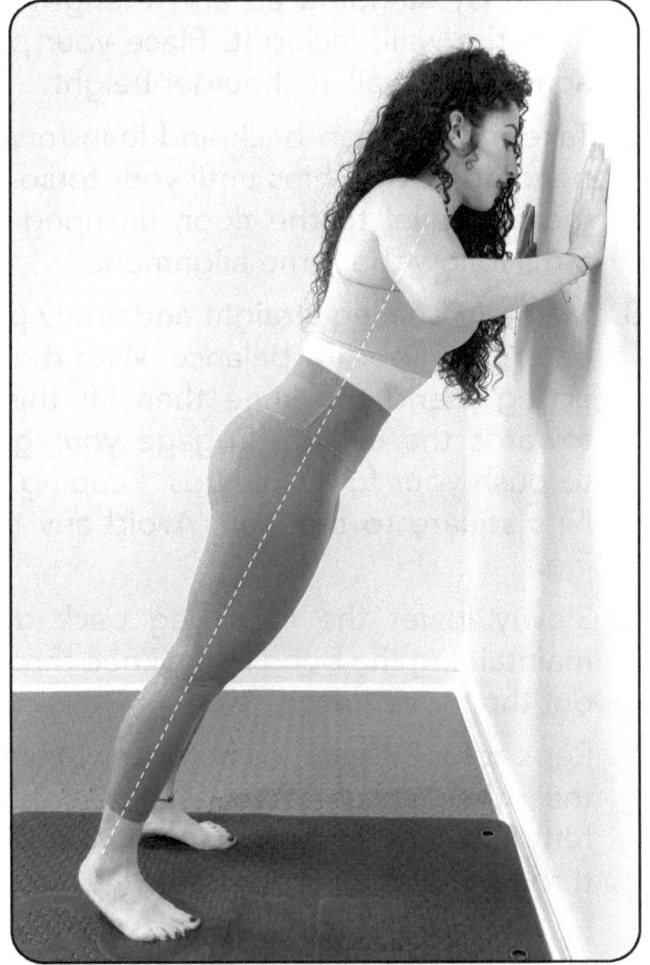

Wall Push-ups are a modified version of traditional push-ups, utilizing a wall to decrease intensity and provide support. This exercise targets the chest, shoulders, and triceps, making it ideal for beginners or those with limited upper body strength. Wall Push-ups effectively improve upper body strength and enhance posture. Additionally, they offer a safe and accessible way to build foundational fitness and promote muscular endurance.

INSTRUCTIONS

1. Stand facing the wall, an arm's length away. Place your palms flat against the wall at shoulder level, slightly wider than shoulder-width apart.

2. As you inhale, lean forward and bend your elbows to lower your body towards the wall, aiming to lightly touch your nose to it, ensuring controlled descent.

3. Keep your body in a straight line, engaging your core to prevent sagging or arching your back.

4. Exhale as you push back, straightening your elbows to return to the starting position.

5. Focus on smooth, controlled motions and rhythmic breathing.

✓ TIPS

- Adjust your starting distance from the wall to alter the difficulty level. The farther you stand, the more intense the exercise will be.

- Focus on engaging your core and glutes throughout the exercise to maximize benefits and protect your lower back.

✗ MISTAKES TO AVOID

- **Locking Elbows:** Avoid completely locking your elbows at the top of the push-up to prevent joint strain.

- **Dropping the Head:** Maintain a neutral neck position by directing your gaze slightly downward.

- **Arching the Back:** Keep your spine neutral throughout the exercise to prevent lower back discomfort.

WALL NARROW PUSH-UPS

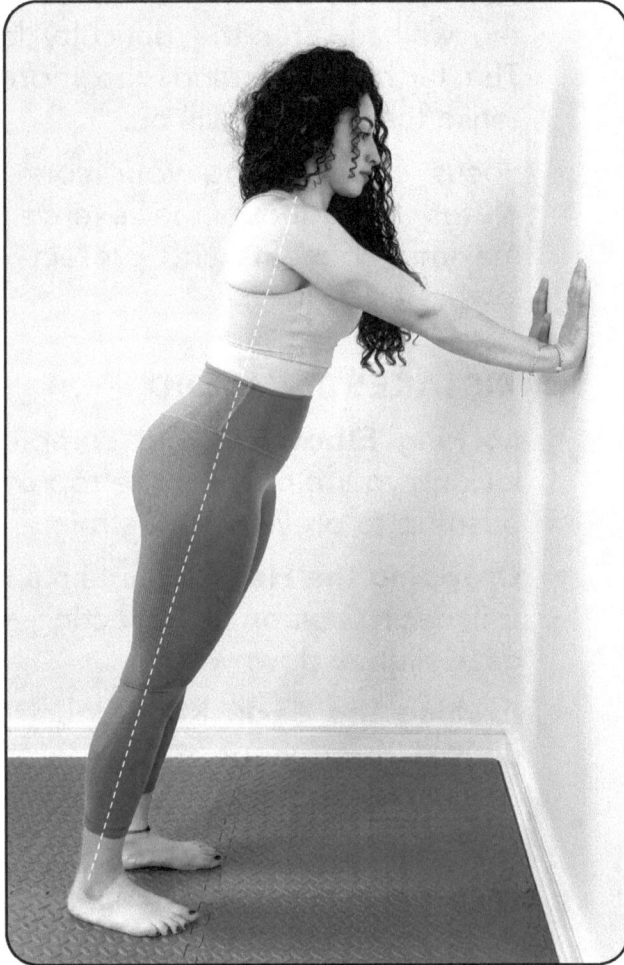

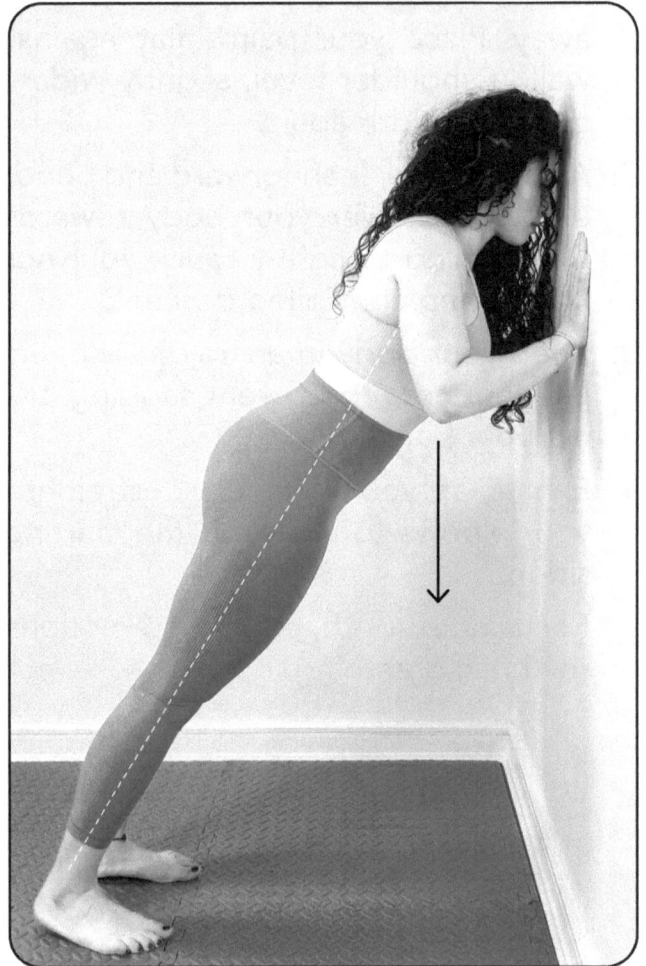

Wall Narrow Push-ups are a specialized variation of the classic push-up, designed to target the triceps and the inner chest by maintaining elbows close to the body. The support from the wall decreases the intensity of the exercise, making it accessible for beginners, those building upper body strength, or individuals focusing on their triceps and inner chest. Additionally, Wall Narrow Push-ups enhance upper body strength and core stability.

INSTRUCTIONS

1. Stand about an arm's length from the wall, facing it. Position your palms on the wall below shoulder level. Keep your elbows pointing towards the floor throughout the exercise.

2. Ensure your elbows point downward towards the floor.

3. Inhale as you lean in, bending your elbows to bring your body closer to the wall. Ensure your elbows remain close to your sides and don't flare out. Try to go as low as possible, lightly touching your forehead to the wall while engaging your core to maintain a straight line from head to heels.

4. Exhale as you press through your palms, straightening your arms to return to the starting position.

5. Continue the exercise for 30 seconds or a set number of repetitions. Focus on the quality of each push-up over speed to prevent injuries and maximize the exercise's effectiveness.

✓ TIPS

- Hold the position close to the wall for one or two seconds on each rep to intensify the tricep engagement.

- Synchronize your breathing with your movements: exhale when pushing away from the wall and inhale as you return, enhancing the push-ups' power and rhythm.

✗ MISTAKES TO AVOID

- **Flaring Elbows:** Avoid letting your elbows flare out to the sides. Keeping them close to your body targets the triceps more effectively.

- **Arching Your Back:** Maintain a neutral spine throughout the push-up to prevent lower back strain.

- **Locking Your Elbows:** Avoid fully extending your elbows at the top of the push-up to protect your joints from strain.

COBRA PUSH-UPS

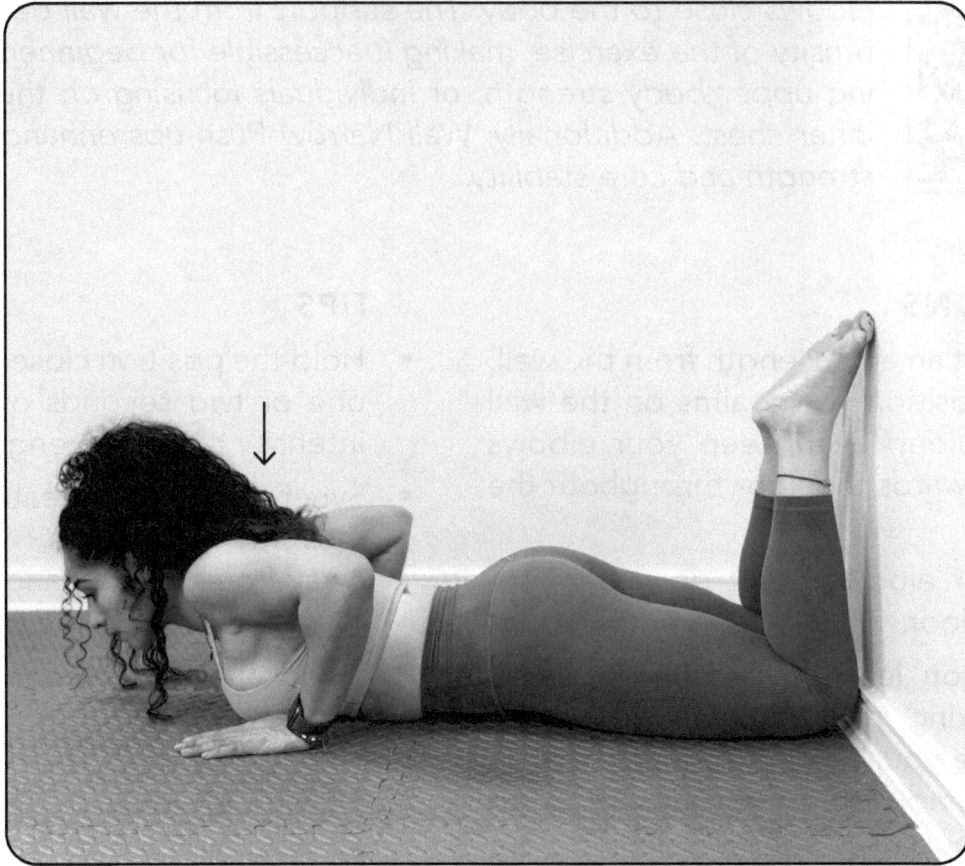

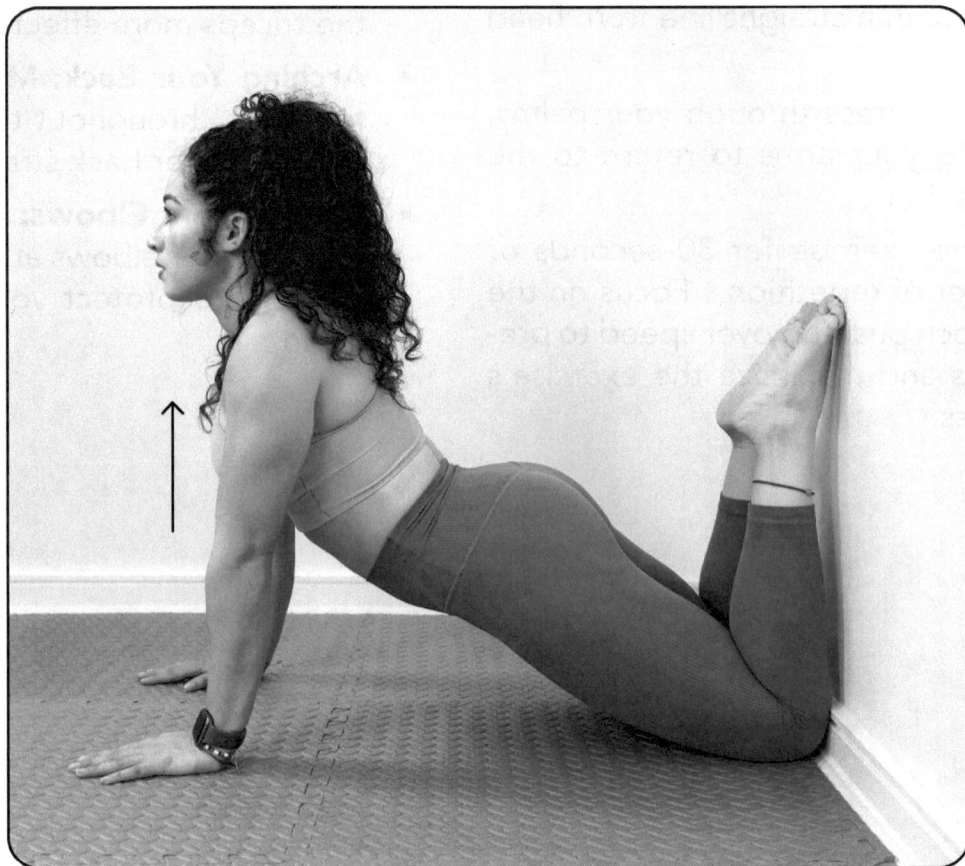

This exercise evolves the traditional cobra stretch into an active Cobra Push-Up, targeting key muscle groups for enhanced strength and control. While the legs remain elevated against the wall, the push-up motion intensifies the workout, engaging the chest, shoulders, and core, without compromising spinal integrity. It's designed to build power and endurance, maintaining a harmonious alignment throughout the body.

INSTRUCTIONS

1. Begin lying face down with your knees at the wall's base and shins extending vertically up the wall.

2. Set your palms flat on the floor directly under your shoulders, bending your elbows close to your sides.

3. Inhale deeply, and as you exhale, press firmly into your palms, lifting your chest and hips off the floor as high as comfortably. Keep your core engaged to avoid straining.

4. Inhale as you gently lower your body back down to the starting position, maintaining control and alignment throughout the movement.

5. Perform for 30 seconds, moving smoothly between the lifted and lowered positions, maintaining a consistent pace and controlled movement.

✓ TIPS

- Focus on engaging your core throughout the exercise to support your lower back.

- Coordinate your breath with your movements—inhale while lowering and exhale while lifting—to optimize oxygen flow and muscle function.

- Keep your gaze down or slightly forward to maintain a neutral neck alignment.

✗ MISTAKES TO AVOID

- **Dropping the Hips:** Avoid letting your hips sag towards the floor. They should lift with your torso to maintain proper alignment and engagement.

- **Flaring the Elbows:** Keep your elbows close to your sides. Flaring them out can put unnecessary stress on your shoulders and reduce the efficacy of the exercise.

- **Overarching Your Back:** While the Wall Cobra Stretch encourages neck and back arching towards your feet, the Wall Cobra Push-ups aim to build muscle strength and endurance without stretching the back. Keep a neutral neck and spine alignment, engaging your core to avoid overarching your lower back during the lift.

SHOULDER PRESS + ALT HEELS

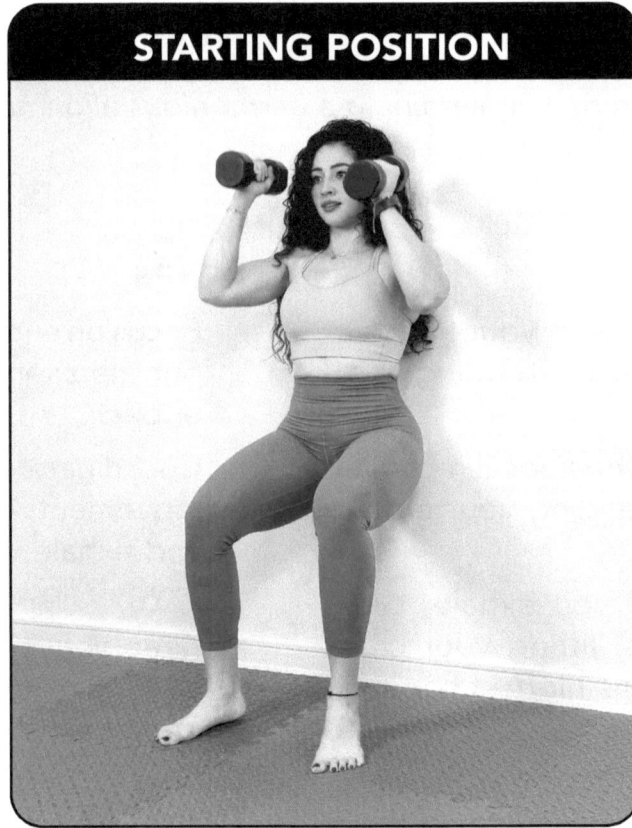
STARTING POSITION

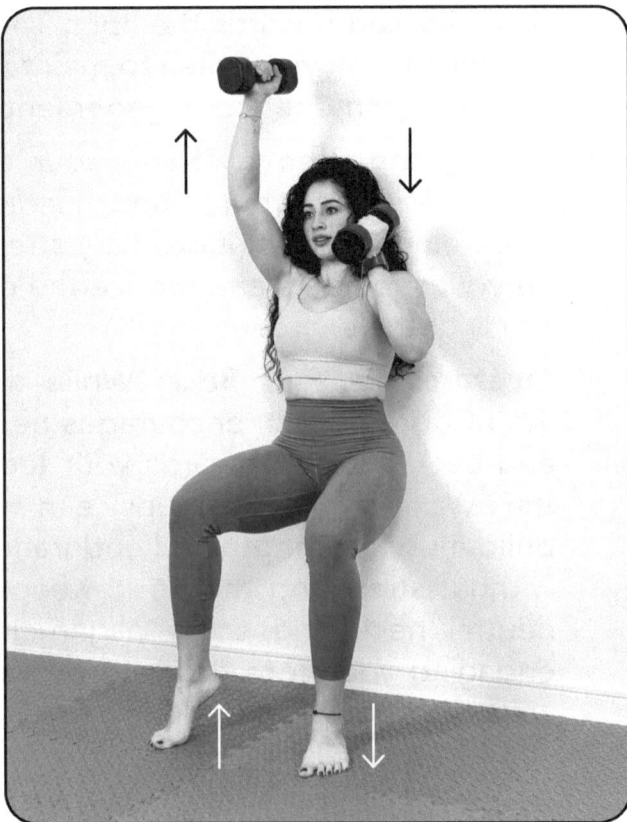

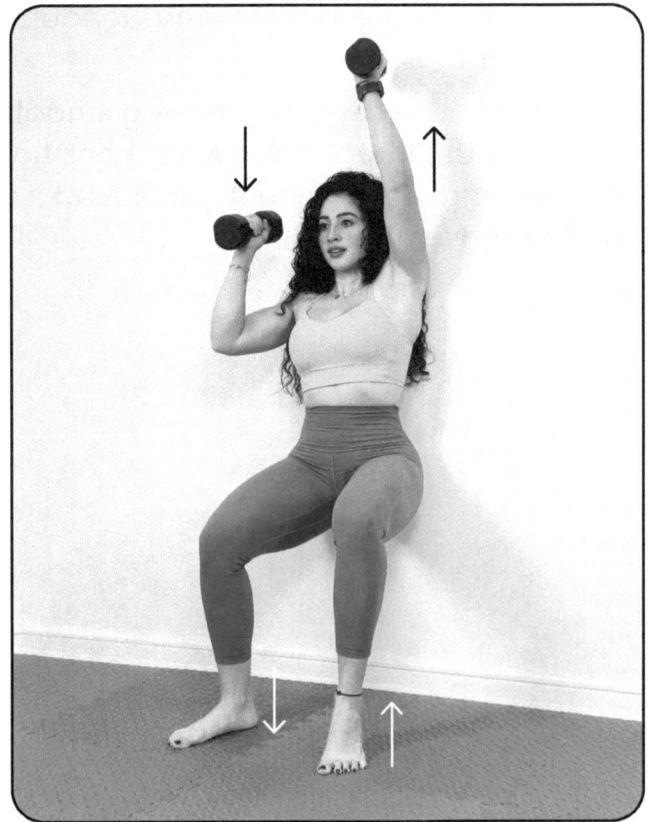

The Shoulder Press with Alternated Heels on the wall is a dynamic exercise that combines lower body stability with upper body strength. By engaging in a wall sit while performing an alternating shoulder press, this exercise targets the shoulders, triceps, quadriceps, and core, providing a comprehensive workout that enhances balance, coordination, and overall body strength.

INSTRUCTIONS

1. Hold a light dumbbell in each hand, or substitute with water bottles or cans. Stand with your back against the wall and slide down into a wall sit position, ensuring your thighs are parallel to the floor.

2. With your back and shoulders against the wall, raise the dumbbells to shoulder height, palms facing each other.

3. As you press one dumbbell overhead, simultaneously lift the heel on the same side. Keep your core engaged and ensure stable posture against the wall.

4. After extending one arm fully (without locking the elbow), bring both the arm and heel back down in a controlled manner. Then, switch to the other arm and heel, maintaining a smooth and steady pace.

5. Alternate arms and heels for the desired number of sets or duration, focusing on maintaining form and balance throughout the exercise.

✓ TIPS

- Coordinate your breath with your movements, exhaling as you press the dumbbell overhead and inhaling as you return to the starting position.

- Maintain your abdominal muscles tight throughout the exercise to support your back and enhance stability.

X MISTAKES TO AVOID

- **Locking the Elbows:** Avoid locking your elbows at the top of the press; keep them slightly bent to maintain tension in the shoulder muscles and protect the joint.

- **Using Heavy Weights:** Do not use weights that are too heavy for this exercise, as it could compromise your form and lead to injury. Light weights are sufficient to provide an effective workout.

- **Leaning Forward:** Keep your back against the wall throughout the exercise to ensure proper form and prevent leaning forward.

CHEST PRESS BRIDGE

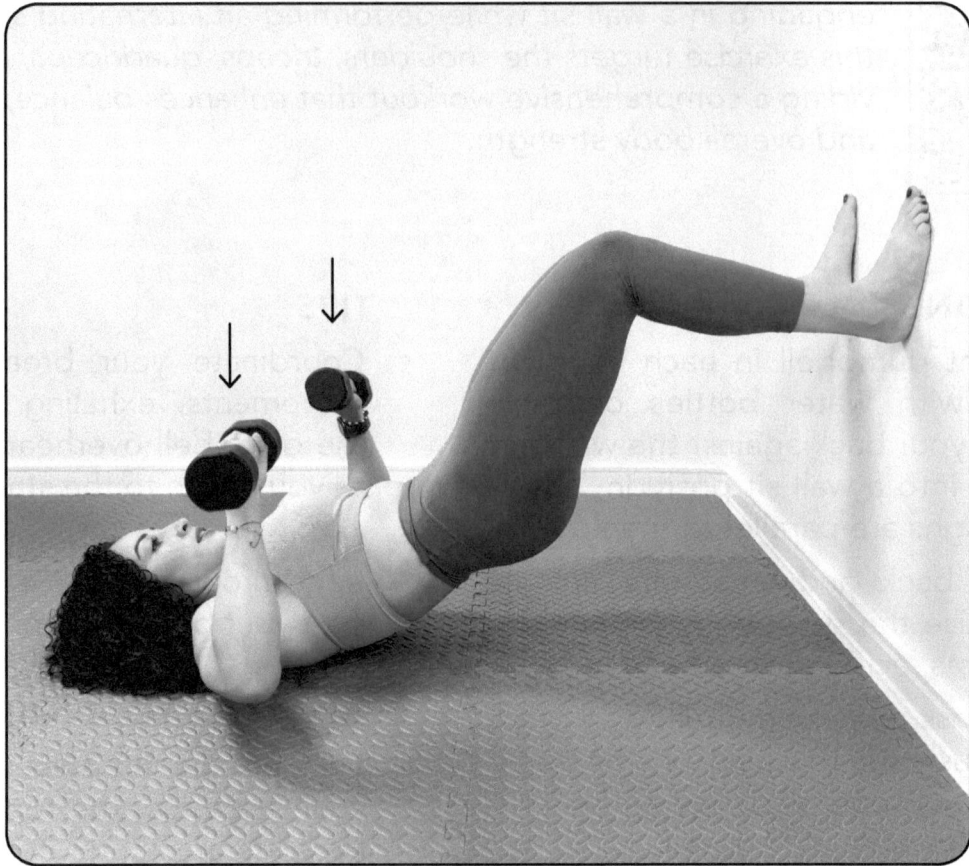

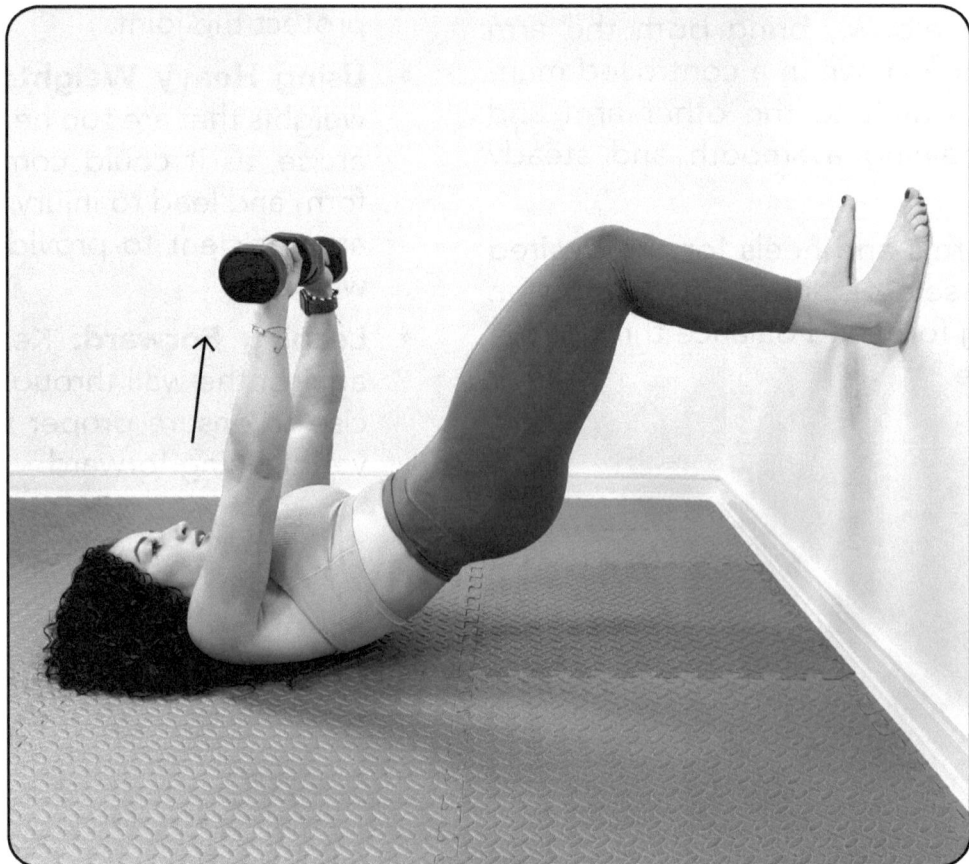

The Chest Press Bridge is an exercise that combines the benefits of a chest press with the core and lower body engagement of a wall bridge. This exercise targets the pectoral muscles, triceps, glutes, and hamstrings, providing a comprehensive workout that enhances upper body strength and improves stability. Performing the chest press in a bridge position increases core activation and encourages more engagement from the lower body, making it an effective full-body exercise.

INSTRUCTIONS

1. Sit on the floor facing the wall with your weights beside you.

2. Lie down on the floor and place your feet on the wall, bending your knees at a 90-degree angle.

3. Grab the dumbbells, one in each hand, and bend your elbows to bring the weights to chest level with your palms facing forward.

4. Engage your core and glutes to lift into the wall bridge position, maintaining the weights at your chest.

5. Once stabilized in the bridge position, press the dumbbells upward, extending your arms fully without locking your elbows. Ensure your wrists remain straight and aligned with your arms.

6. After completing the press, lower the dumbbells back to chest level in a controlled manner.

7. Repeat for 30 seconds.

✓ TIPS

- Ensure your movements are smooth and coordinated, with a focus on maintaining proper form in both the chest press and the bridge.

- Inhale as you lower the weights and exhale as you press them up, coordinating your breathing with your movements.

✗ MISTAKES TO AVOID

- **Wrist Bending:** Maintain straight wrists throughout the exercise to avoid unnecessary pressure and potential strain.

- **Losing Hip Elevation:** Ensure your hips remain lifted and stable throughout the exercise to maximize the effectiveness of the bridge position.

HUG THE TREE

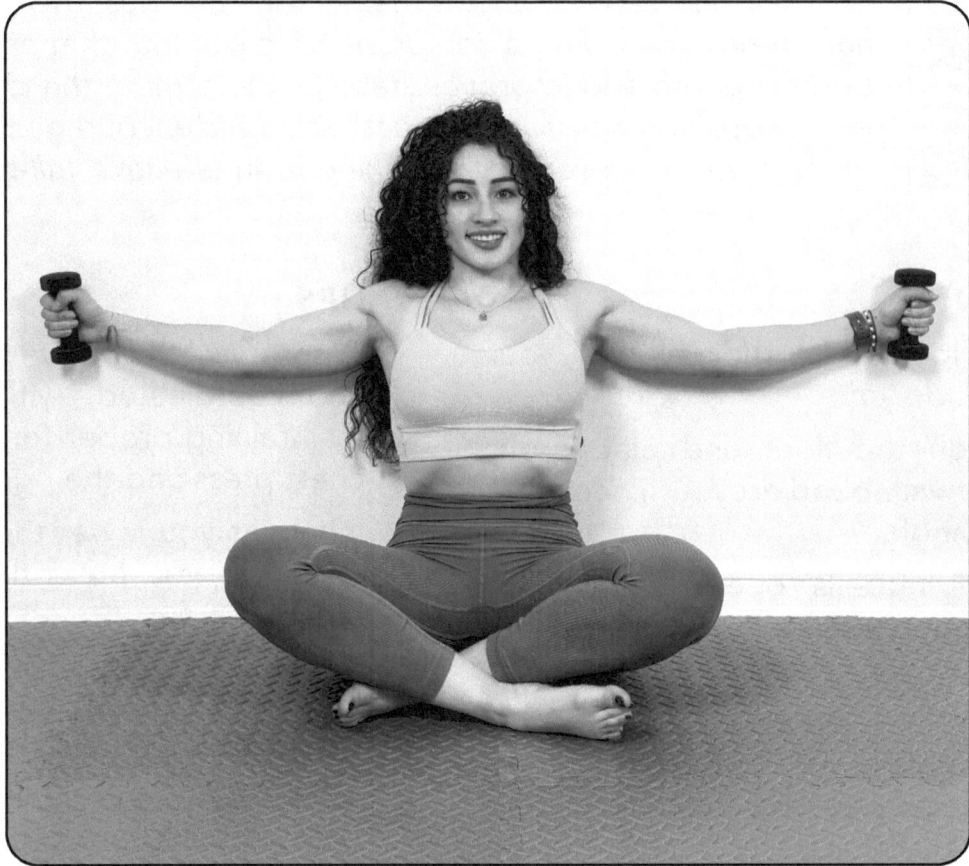

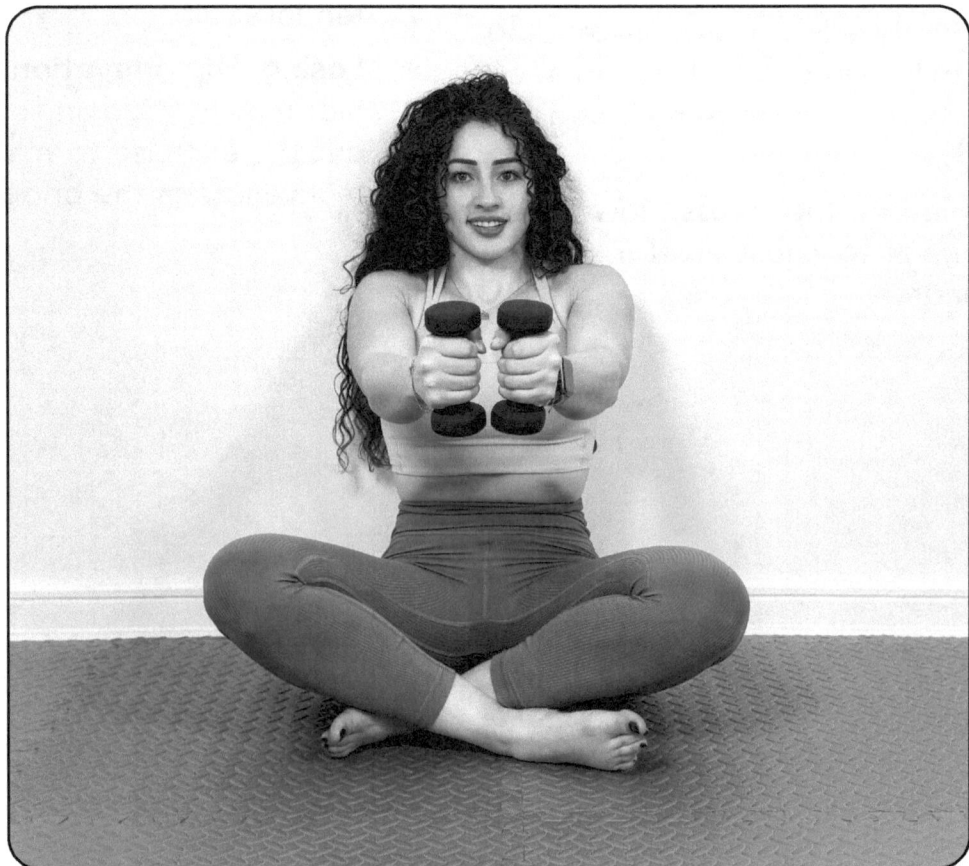

The Hug the Tree exercise performed against the wall is a gentle, yet effective movement that targets the chest, shoulders, and upper back muscles, enhancing strength and promoting better posture. This exercise simulates the action of encircling a large tree with your arms, engaging your upper body in a controlled and mindful manner. By incorporating light dumbbells into the exercise, you not only maintain the engagement of your upper body but also incrementally increase muscle endurance and strength.

INSTRUCTIONS

1. Begin by sitting comfortably on the floor with your back and hips pressed firmly against the wall, holding a dumbbell in each hand.

2. With your arms extended at shoulder height and palms facing forward, hold the dumbbells with a slight bend in your elbows. Make sure your shoulders and neck are relaxed in a neutral position.

3. As you bring your arms together in front of you, mimicking the action of hugging a grand tree, exhale deeply to enhance the engagement of your chest and shoulder muscles.

4. From this position, slowly open your arms back to the starting position, inhale deeply, filling your lungs and expanding your chest, to maximize the stretch and relaxation of the muscles.

5. Continue this exercise, following the rhythm of your breath—inhaling as you open your arms and exhaling as you bring them together—for five complete breaths, ensuring a harmonious blend of movement and breathing for optimal effectiveness. Be mindful to keep your shoulders and back against the wall throughout the entire exercise.

✓ TIPS

- To maximize control and effectiveness, maintain deep, steady breaths in sync with your movements. Ensure each action is slow and smooth, concentrating on relaxation and form.

- For an added challenge, perform this exercise while standing and leaning against the wall in a wall sit position. This variation will engage your core and lower body in addition to your upper body.

✗ MISTAKES TO AVOID

- **Shoulder Misalignment:** Ensure your shoulders don't rise up. A loss of alignment in your shoulders can indicate fatigue, which may suggest the need to reduce the weight you are using.

- **Using Heavy Weights:** Select dumbbells that allow you to maintain proper form throughout the exercise. Heavy weights may cause your shoulders to lose form and assume an incorrect posture.

- **Breaking Wall Contact:** Ensure that your entire back, especially your shoulders, remains in contact with the wall throughout the exercise to maintain proper posture.

SERVE A PLATTER

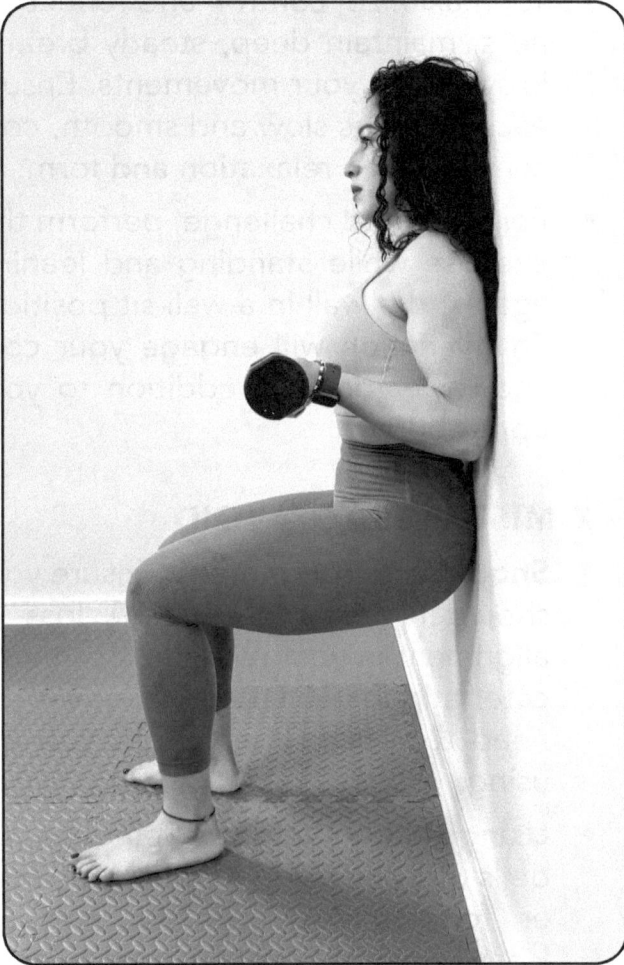

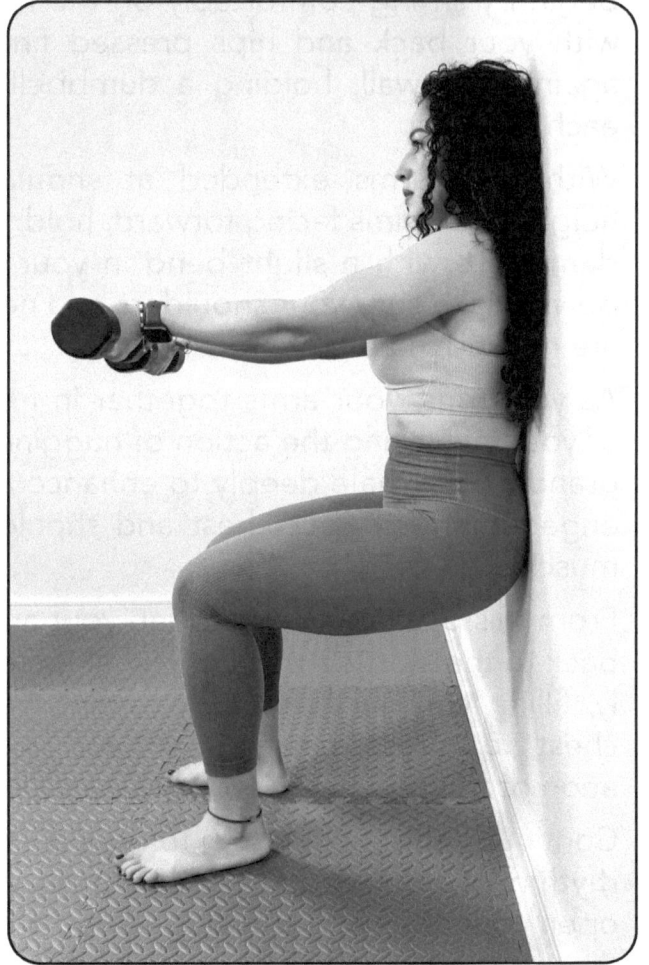

Serve a Platter against the wall is a functional exercise that targets the shoulders and engages the biceps. This exercise simulates the action of serving a platter, helping to improve shoulder stability, coordination and posture. Performing this movement against the wall ensures proper alignment and increases the exercise's effectiveness by providing feedback on your form.

INSTRUCTIONS

1. Grab two light weights, one in each hand, and position yourself with your back and shoulders against the wall. If you are advanced, you can adopt the wall sit position to engage your core and triceps throughout the exercise. Otherwise, you can perform this exercise standing or comfortably sitting on the floor, as long as your back doesn't arch and remains in contact with the wall.

2. Extend your arms in front of you at shoulder height, palms facing up as if holding a platter. Keep a slight bend in your elbows to avoid stress on the joints.

3. Once your arms are fully extended, hold the position for a moment, then slowly return to the starting position, maintaining the alignment of your back against the wall.

4. Repeat the exercise for 30 seconds, focusing on the precision of the movement and the stability of your shoulders and back.

✓ TIP

- Coordinate your breathing with the movement. Exhale from your mouth when pushing your arms forward, and inhale through your nose when bringing your arms back.

✗ MISTAKES TO AVOID

- **Shoulder Misalignment:** Avoid letting your shoulders elevate or round forward. Bring them back against the wall, keeping your chest as open as possible.

- **Using Heavy Weights:** Using heavy weights can compromise form, causing improper alignment and reducing muscle engagement. Opt for weights that allow you to maintain proper posture and control.

- **Breaking Wall Contact:** Ensure that your shoulders and lower back remain in contact with the wall throughout the exercise to maintain proper posture and effectiveness.

SKULL CRUSHERS

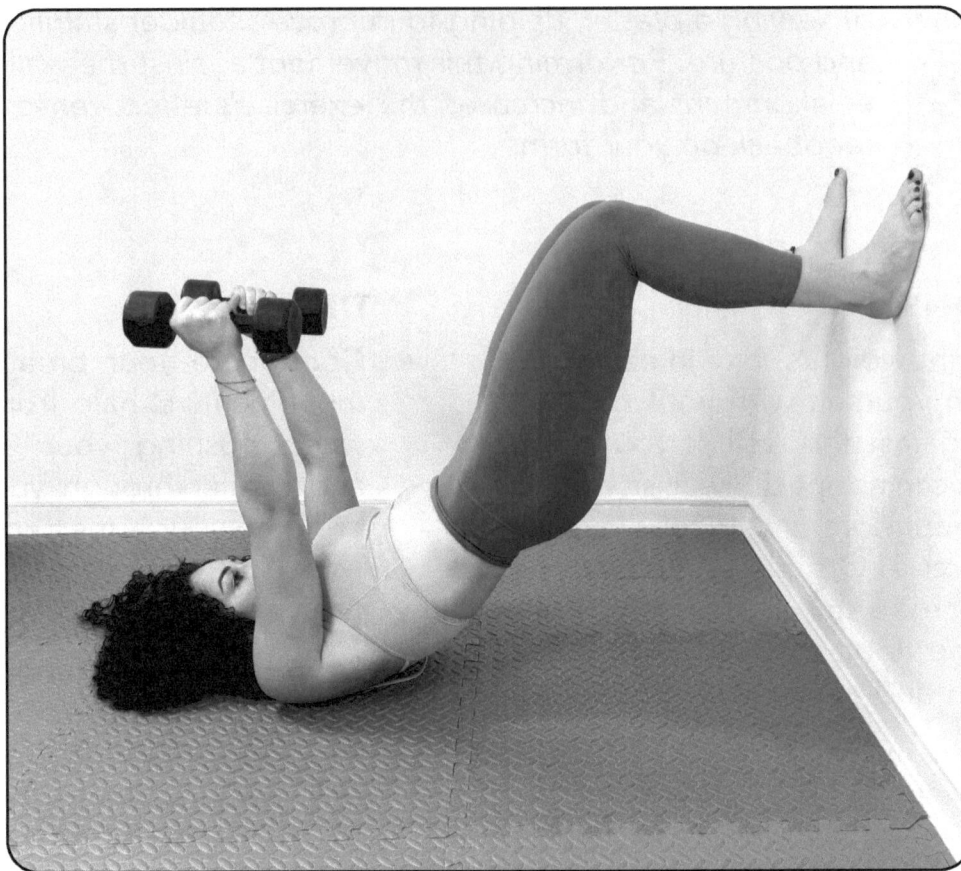

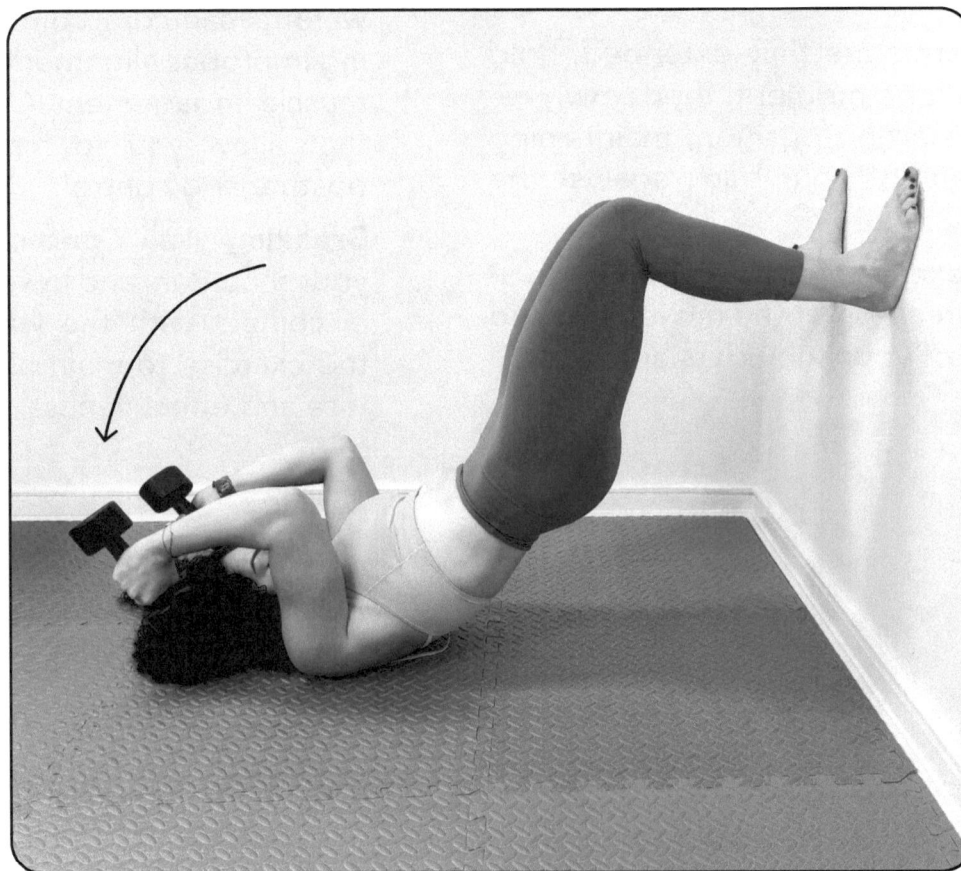

The Skull Crushers exercise in a wall bridge position is a variation that targets the triceps muscles while also engaging the core and glutes for necessary stability. This exercise enriches the classic skullcrusher with added intensity from the wall-supported bridge, offering an effective full-body workout that boosts upper arm strength and core stability.

INSTRUCTIONS

1. Begin by sitting on the floor facing the wall with your weights beside you.

2. Lie down and place your feet flat against the wall with knees bent.

3. Press your feet into the wall to lift your hips up, entering into a bridge position.

4. With hips elevated, extend your arms above your chest holding the dumbbells, palms facing each other.

5. Bend your elbows, lowering the dumbbells toward your forehead, keeping upper arms still and elbows pointed upwards in a controlled motion.

6. Extend your arms, lifting the dumbbells to the starting position, concentrating on engaging the triceps and maintaining core and glute activation.

7. Continue for 30 seconds or the desired number of repetitions, keeping consistent with the bridge posture and tricep focus.

✓ TIP

- Inhale while lowering the dumbbells and exhale when extending your arms, syncing your breath with your movements for better focus and stability.

✗ MISTAKES TO AVOID

- **Flaring Elbows:** Keep your elbows tucked in, aligned above your shoulders, to focus the effort on your triceps and avoid joint stress.

- **Losing Hip Elevation:** Consistently monitor your bridge position to prevent hip sagging, maintaining exercise effectiveness and protecting your lower back.

- **Overloading Weights:** Using weights beyond your capacity can compromise your technique and strain your muscles. Select weights that allows you to complete each set with proper form and full control.

SIT & TWIST

STARTING POSITION

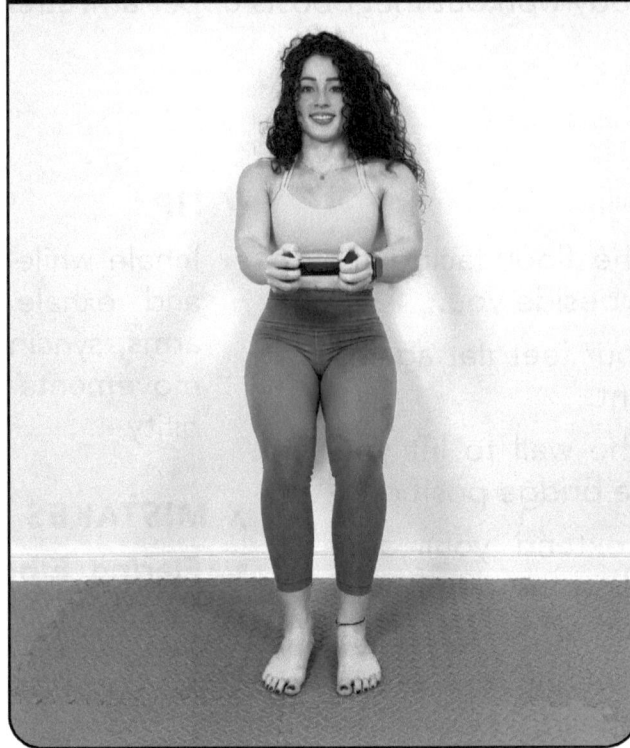

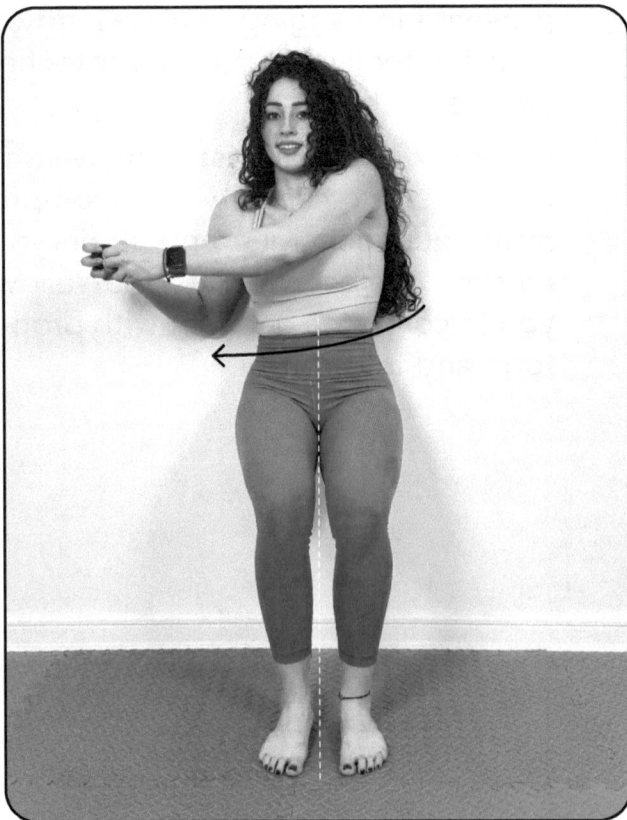

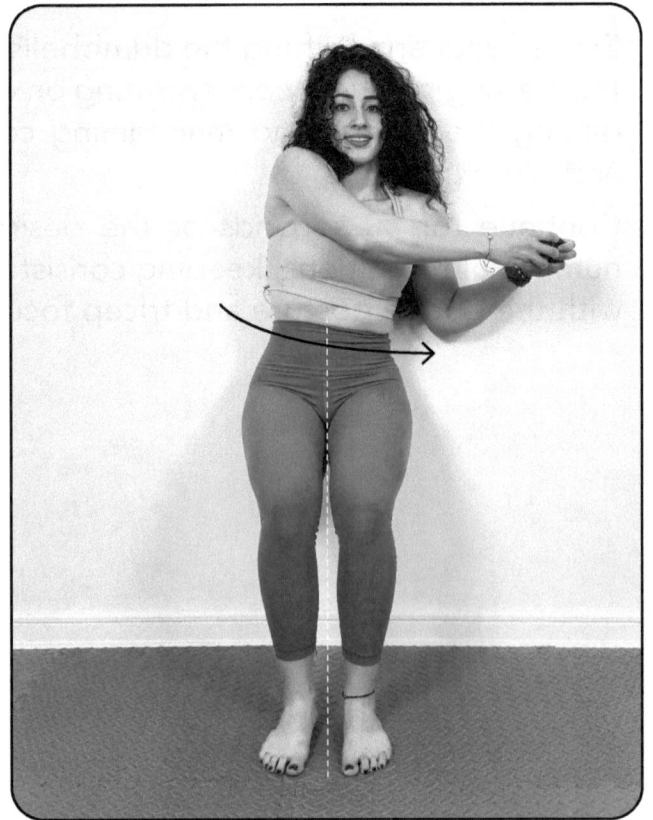

The Sit & Twist exercise performed against the wall is an excellent movement targeting the oblique muscles, enhancing core stability and rotational strength. Using one weight, this exercise also engages the shoulders and arms, providing a comprehensive upper body workout. The support from the wall helps ensure proper posture and alignment throughout the movement, maximizing the effectiveness of the twist and engaging the core muscles deeply.

INSTRUCTIONS

1. Sit against the wall with your back and hips pressed firmly against the wall and your legs extended in front of you. Hold a dumbbell or a suitable weight with both hands in front of your chest, with your arms bent at approximately 90 degrees.

2. While keeping your back flat against the wall, rotate your torso to one side, guiding the weight toward the outside of your hip. Ensure this twisting motion is controlled and originates from your core, not your arms.

3. Slowly bring your torso and the weight back to the center, then execute the twist to the other side with the same controlled, deliberate motion, ensuring your back stays pressed against the wall.

4. Repeat for 30 seconds, focusing on the precision of each twist while ensuring your posture remains intact against the wall. Conclude the exercise by bringing the weight back to the center position.

✓ TIP

- Keep your spine long and back pressed firmly against the wall throughout the exercise to ensure proper alignment and maximize the oblique engagement.

✗ MISTAKES TO AVOID

- **Slouching:** Avoid letting your back round or come off the wall, which can reduce the engagement of the core.

- **Using Momentum:** Maintain a slow and controlled movement speed to increase the effectiveness of the twist and prevent momentum from reducing the workout's intensity.

- **Overreaching:** Do not twist too far or with too much force, as this can compromise your balance and strain your back. Ensure the movement is within a comfortable range.

- **Gripping the Weight Too Tightly:** Maintain a firm but relaxed grip on the weight to prevent unnecessary tension in your arms and shoulders.

WORKOUTS AND ROUTINES

Welcome to the Workouts and Routines chapter, where we delve into wall pilates workouts that build upon the exercises detailed in the previous chapter. This section offers three types of routines: Stretching (aimed at enhancing flexibility and reducing muscle soreness), Posture Improvement (designed to align and stretch your spine while strengthening the key muscles that support and enhance good posture), and Muscle Toning (focused on firming and sculpting specific muscle groups: arms, legs, core, or the entire body).

Each workout spans 3 to 6 minutes to accommodate even the busiest schedules. We suggest pairing a Muscle Toning routine with a Stretching routine to craft a comprehensive 10-minute training session. These workouts serve as a foundation—feel free to mix and match the wall pilates exercises to tailor routines that align with your goals and preferences.

STRETCHING 1

DURATION:
3 min **30** sec

GOAL:
Flexibility and Pain Relief

1. SPINE EXTENSION
(PAGE 29)

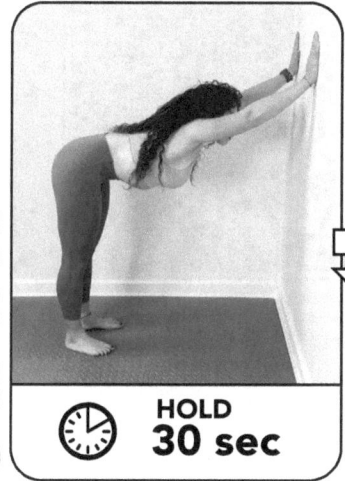

START

HOLD
30 sec

2. SIDE BEND LEFT
(PAGE 18)

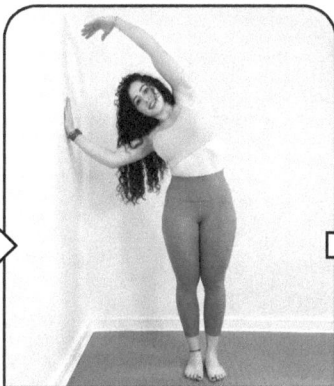

HOLD
30 sec

3. SIDE BEND RIGHT
(PAGE 18)

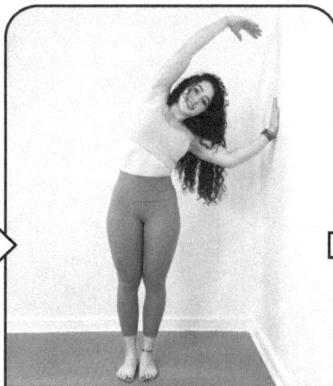

HOLD
30 sec

4. QUAD STRETCH RIGHT LEG (PAGE 15)

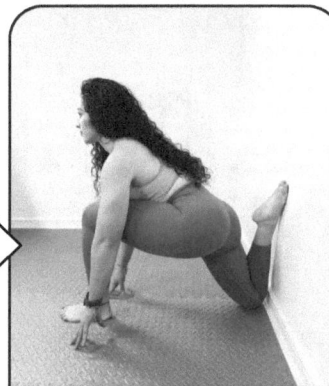

HOLD
30 sec

5. QUAD STRETCH LEFT LEG (PAGE 15)

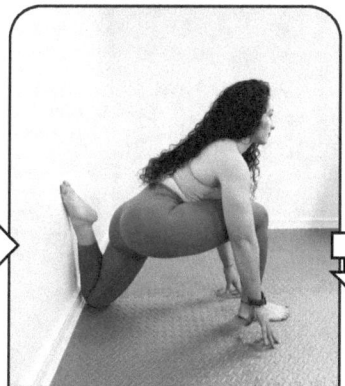

HOLD
30 sec

6. STRADDLE SPLIT
(PAGE 30)

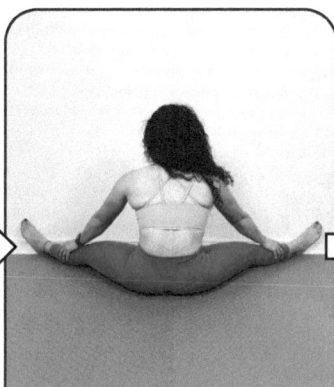

HOLD
30 sec

7. SCISSORS
(PAGE 36)

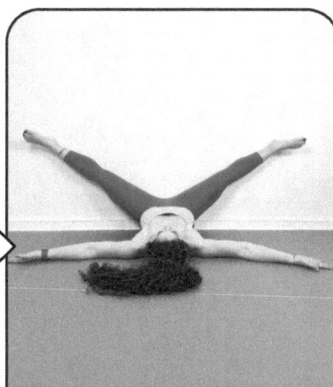

FINISH

30 sec

STRETCHING 2

⏱ **DURATION:**

4 min

🎯 **GOAL:**

Flexibility and Pain Relief

1. SPINE ROTATION ALTERNATE (PAGE 20)

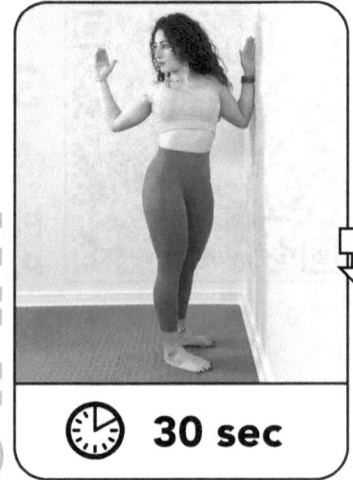

START

⏰ **30 sec**

2. KNEELING T.R. LEFT (PAGE 26)

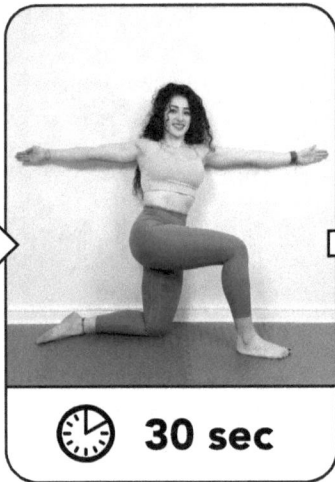

⏰ **30 sec**

3. KNEELING T.R. RIGHT (PAGE 26)

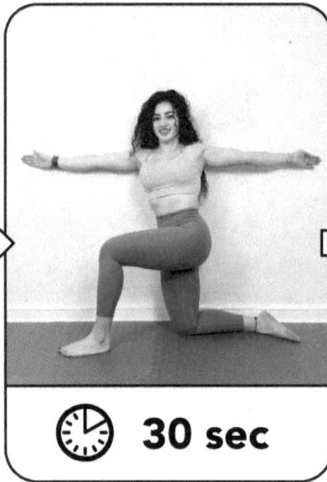

⏰ **30 sec**

4. WALL COBRA (PAGE 28)

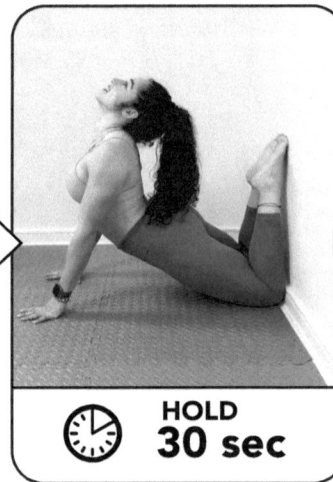

⏰ **HOLD 30 sec**

5. STRADDLE SPLIT SIDE LEFT (PAGE 31)

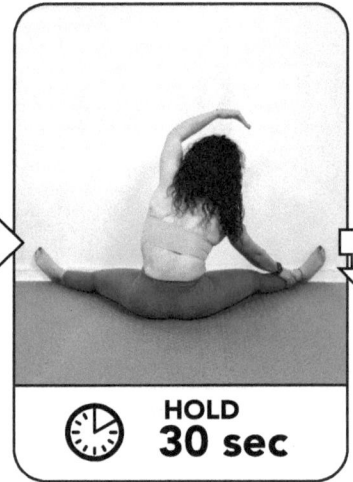

⏰ **HOLD 30 sec**

6. STRADDLE SPLIT SIDE RIGHT (PAGE 31)

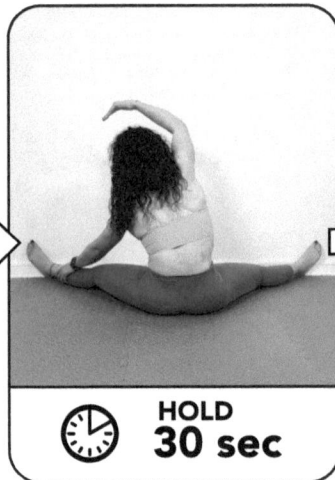

⏰ **HOLD 30 sec**

7. BICEP STRETCH LEFT (PAGE 16)

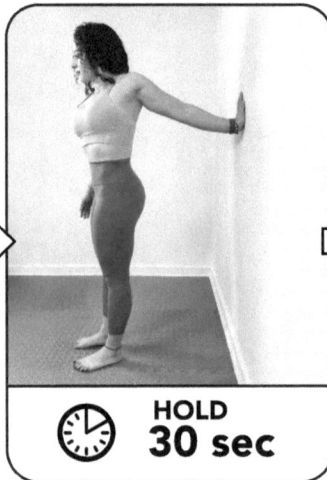

⏰ **HOLD 30 sec**

8. BICEP STRETCH RIGHT (PAGE 16)

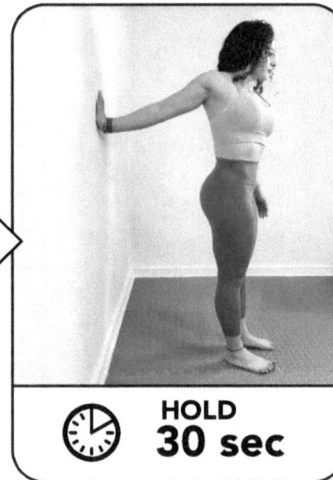

FINISH

⏰ **HOLD 30 sec**

STRETCHING 3

⏱ **DURATION:**
3 min

◎ **GOAL:**
Flexibility and Pain Relief

1. WALL COBRA
(PAGE 28)

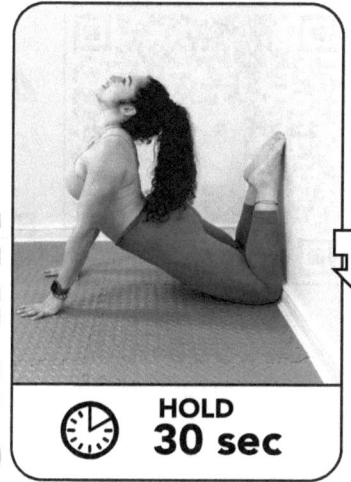

START

🕐 **HOLD**
30 sec

2. WALL BUTTERFLY
(PAGE 32)

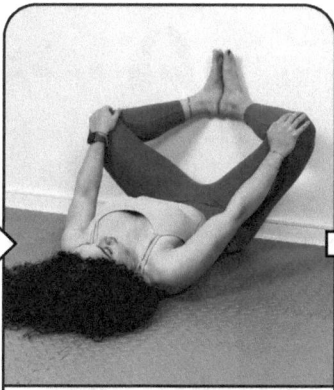

🕐 **HOLD**
30 sec

3. CROSSED LEG S. LEFT (PAGE 33)

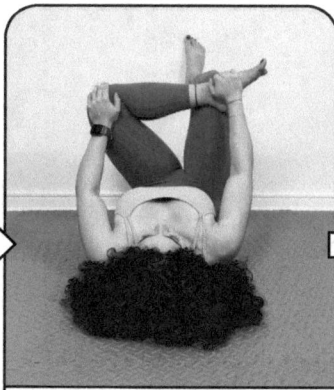

🕐 **HOLD**
30 sec

4. CROSSED LEG S. RIGHT (PAGE 33)

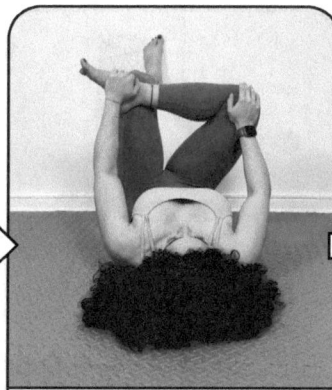

🕐 **HOLD**
30 sec

5. L LEG STRETCHING LEFT (PAGE 34)

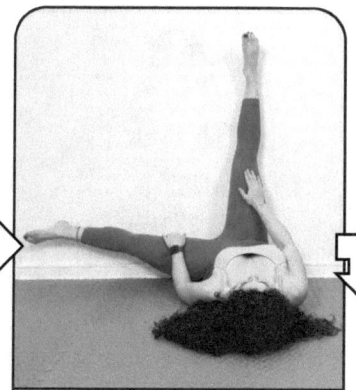

🕐 **HOLD**
30 sec

6. L LEG STRETCHING RIGHT (PAGE 34)

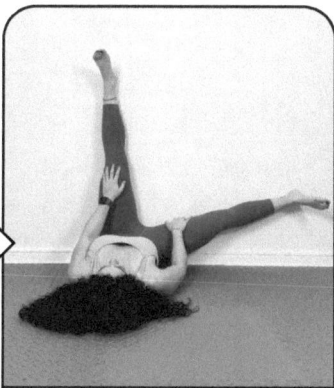

FINISH

🕐 **HOLD**
30 sec

POSTURE IMPROVEMENT 1

DURATION:
4 min

GOAL:
Better Posture

1. WALL SCARECROW ROTATIONS (PAGE 24)

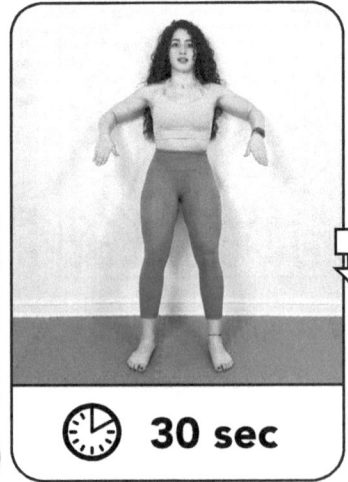

START

🕐 **30 sec**

2. WALL ANGEL
(PAGE 22)

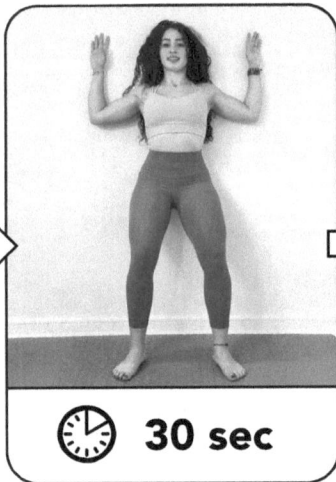

🕐 **30 sec**

3. SERVE A PLATTER
(PAGE 82)

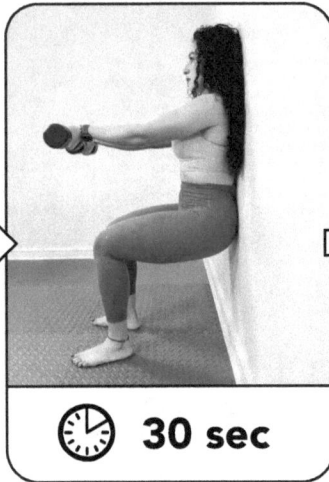

🕐 **30 sec**

4. REST

🕐 **30 sec**

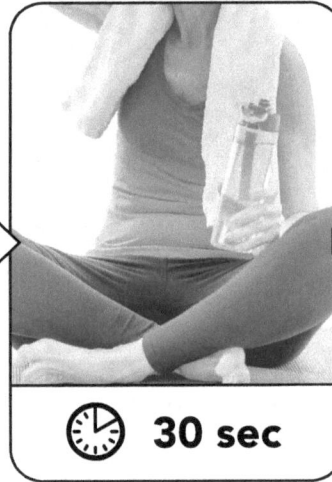

5. WALL SCARECROW ROTATIONS (PAGE 24)

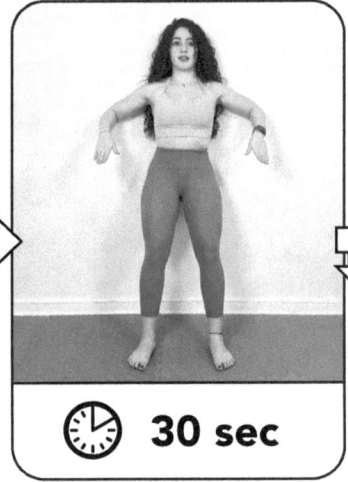

🕐 **30 sec**

6. HUG THE TREE
(PAGE 80)

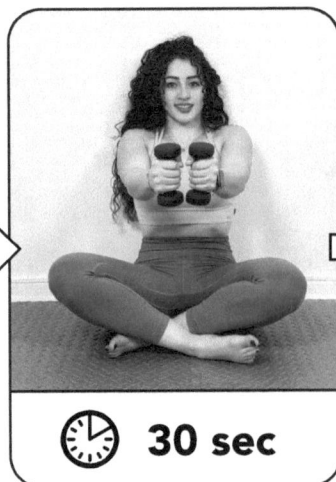

🕐 **30 sec**

7. KNEELING T.R. LEFT
(PAGE 26)

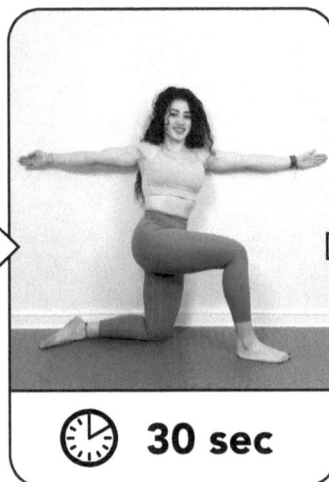

🕐 **30 sec**

8. KNEELING T.R. RIGHT (PAGE 26)

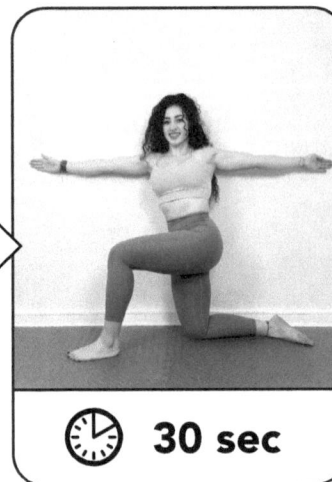

FINISH

🕐 **30 sec**

POSTURE IMPROVEMENT 2

DURATION:

4 min

GOAL:

Better Posture

1. HUG THE TREE
(PAGE 80)

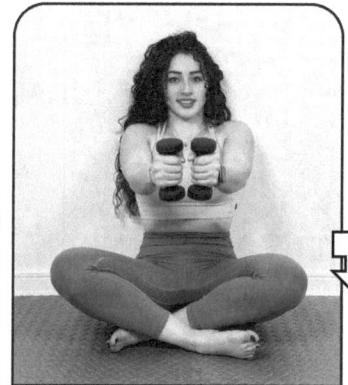

START

🕐 **30 sec**

---

2. WALL ANGEL
(PAGE 22)

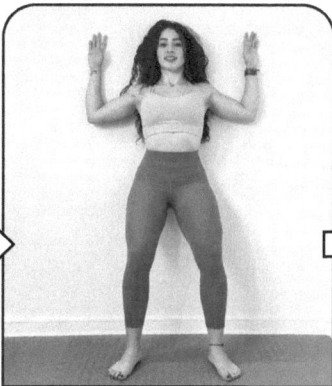

🕐 **30 sec**

3. REST

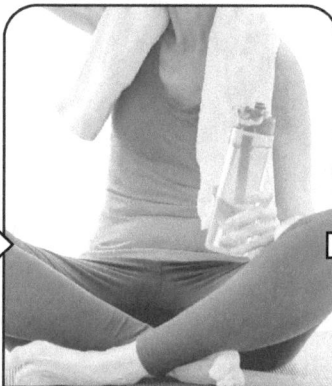

🕐 **30 sec**

4. SERVE A PLATTER
(PAGE 82)

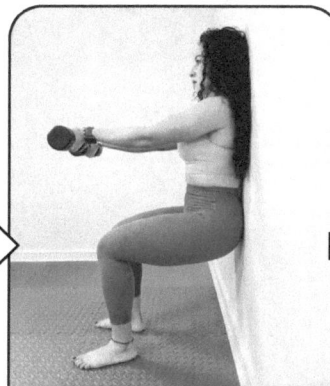

🕐 **30 sec**

5. HUG THE TREE
(PAGE 80)

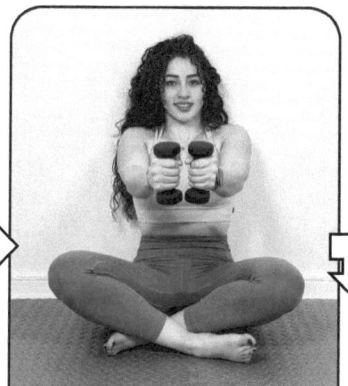

🕐 **30 sec**

---

6. REST

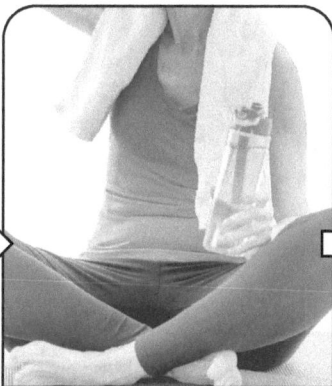

🕐 **30 sec**

7. WALL SCARECROW
ROTATIONS (PAGE 24)

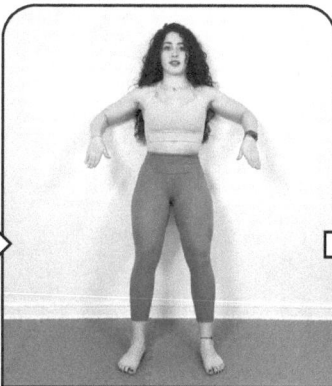

🕐 **30 sec**

8. WALL SIT
(PAGE 12)

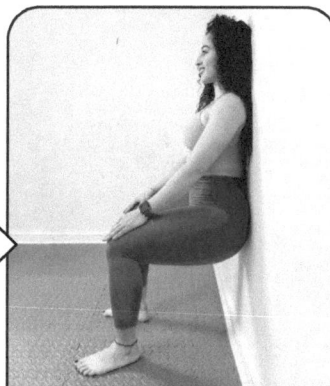

FINISH

🕐 **HOLD 30 sec**

MUSCLE TONING - LEGS 1

⏱ **DURATION:**
4 min **30** sec

🎯 **GOAL:**
Leg Muscle Toning and Flexibility

1. WALL SIT
(PAGE 12)

2. SIDE LEG RAISES
LEFT (PAGE 17)

START

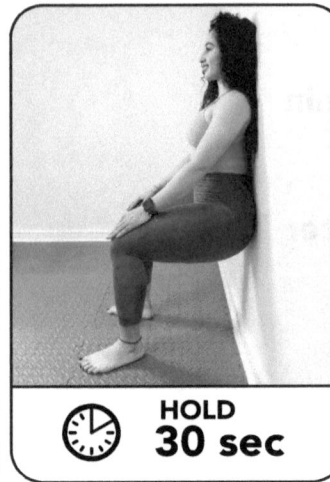

HOLD
30 sec

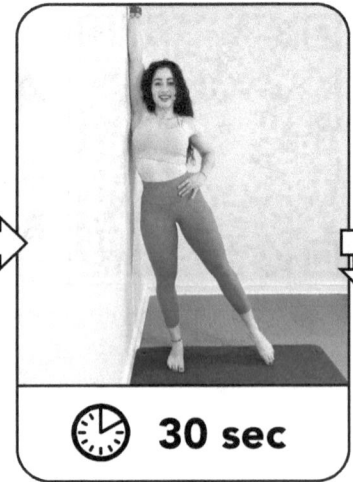

30 sec

3. SIDE LEG RAISES
RIGHT (PAGE 17)

4. REST

5. WALL SIT HEEL
RAISE (PAGE 13)

6. KICKBACK HOLD
LEFT (PAGE 41)

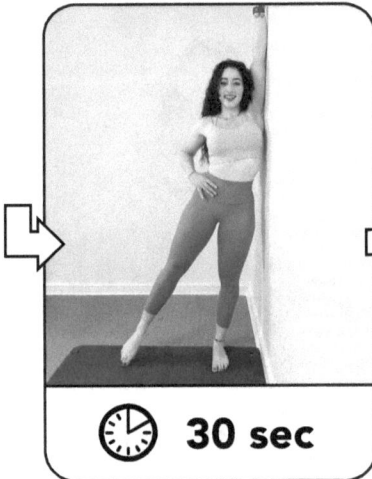

30 sec

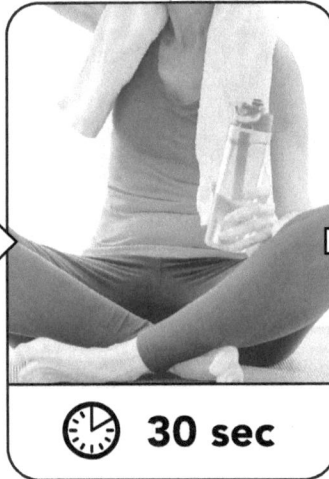

30 sec

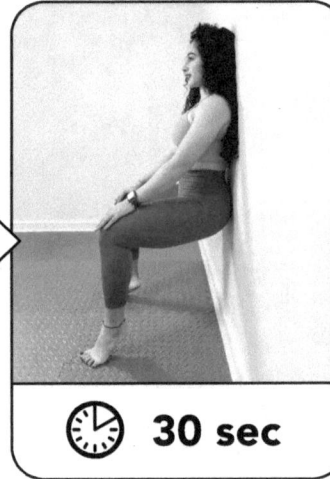

30 sec

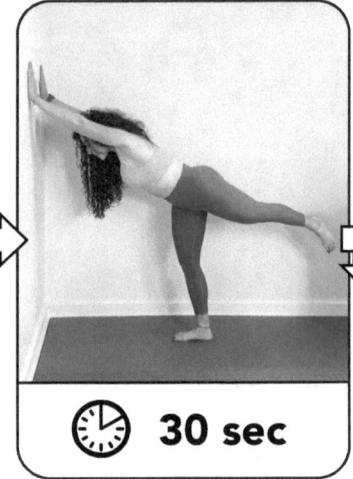

30 sec

7. KICKBACK HOLD
RIGHT (PAGE 41)

8. HIP LIFTS
(PAGE 38)

9. WALL-SUPPORTED
KNEE RAISE (P. 66)

FINISH

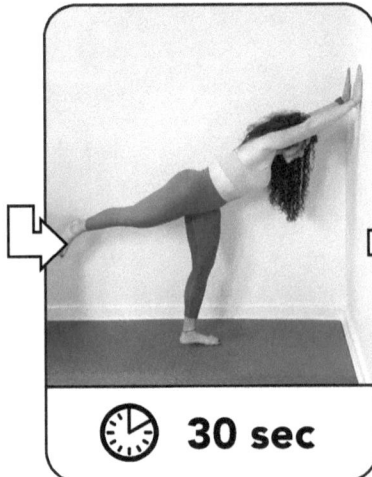

30 sec

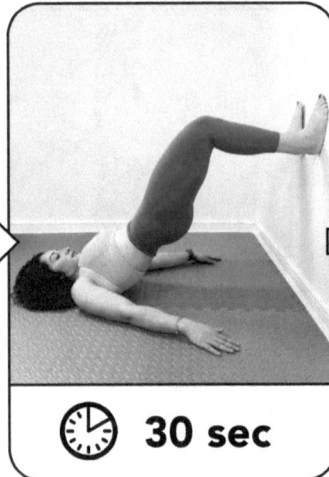

30 sec

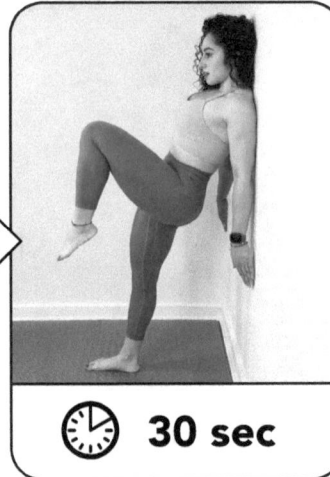

30 sec

MUSCLE TONING - LEGS 2

DURATION:
5 min

GOAL:
Muscle Toning, Endurance and Flexibility

START

1. W.S. DONKEY KICK LEFT (PAGE 68)
30 sec

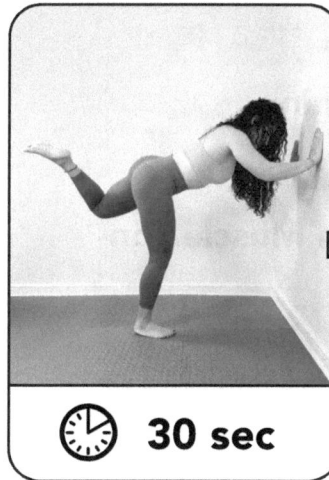

2. W.S. DONKEY KICK RIGHT (PAGE 68)
30 sec

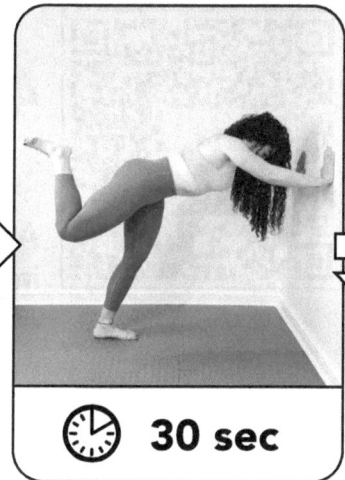

3. KICKBACK HOLD LEFT (PAGE 41)
30 sec

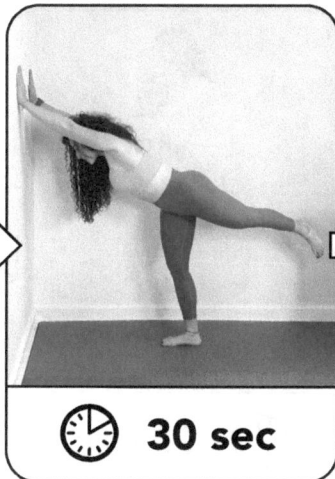

4. KICKBACK HOLD RIGHT (PAGE 41)
30 sec

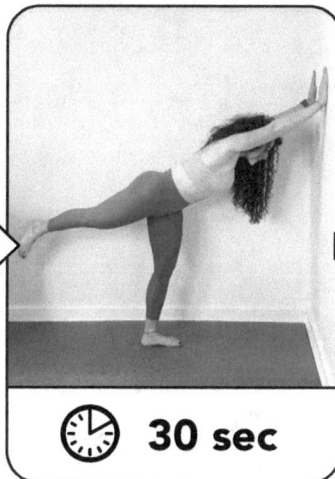

5. WALL SIT (PAGE 12)
HOLD 30 sec

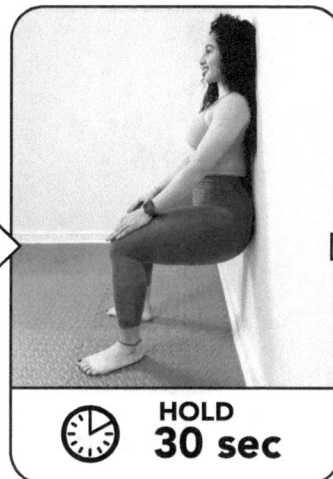

6. REST
30 sec

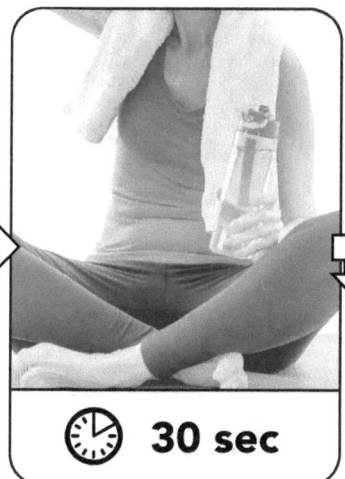

7. WALL SIT HEEL RAISE (PAGE 13)
30 sec

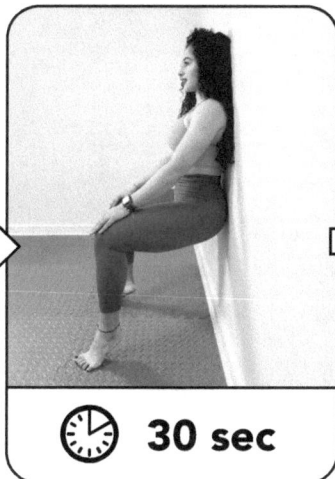

8. SIDE LEG RAISES LEFT (PAGE 17)
30 sec

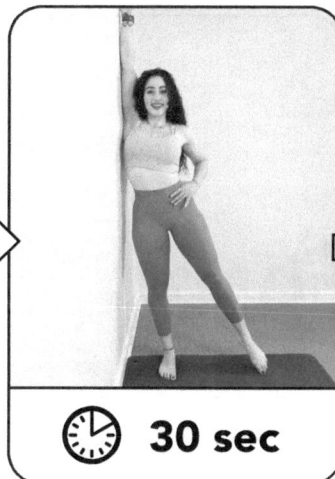

9. SIDE LEG RAISES RIGHT (PAGE 17)
30 sec

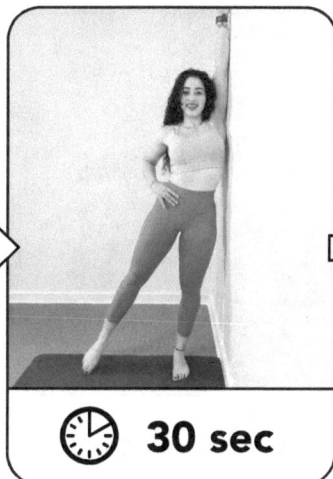

10. WALL-SUPPORTED KNEE RAISE (PAGE 66)
30 sec

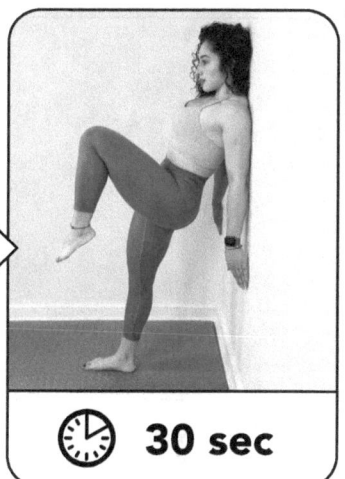

FINISH

MUSCLE TONING - ARMS 1

DURATION:

4 min

GOAL:

Arm Muscle Toning

1. WALL PUSH-UPS
(PAGE 70)

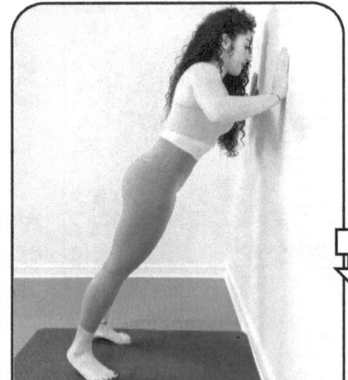

START

🕐 **30 sec**

2. SERVE A PLATTER
(PAGE 82)

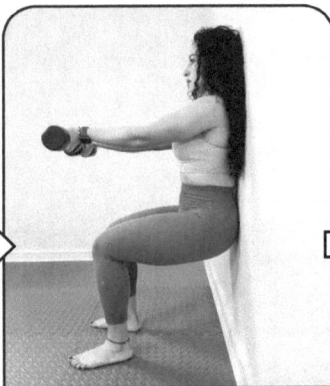

🕐 **30 sec**

3. SHOULDER TAPS
(PAGE 52)

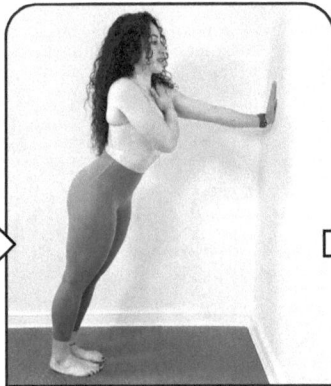

🕐 **30 sec**

4. REST

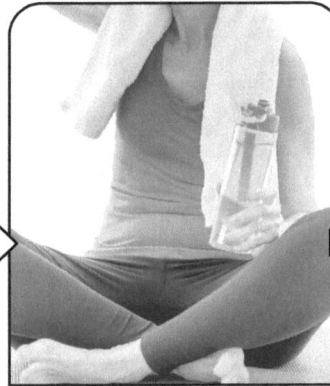

🕐 **30 sec**

5. WALL PLANK UPS
(PAGE 50)

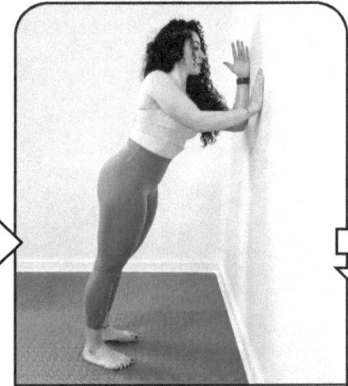

🕐 **30 sec**

6. SHOULDER PRESS + ALT HEELS (PAGE 76)

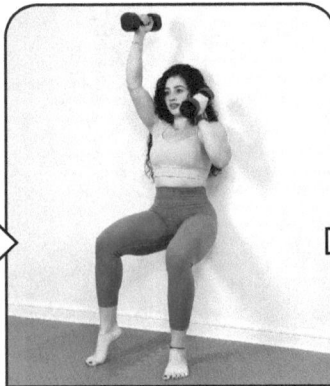

🕐 **30 sec**

7. CHEST PRESS BRIDGE (PAGE 78)

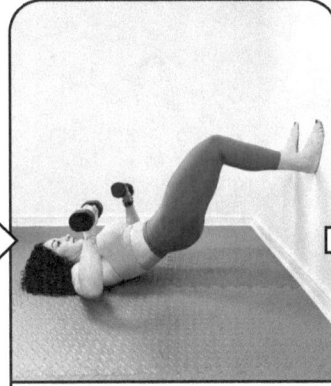

🕐 **30 sec**

8. SKULL CRUSHERS
(PAGE 84)

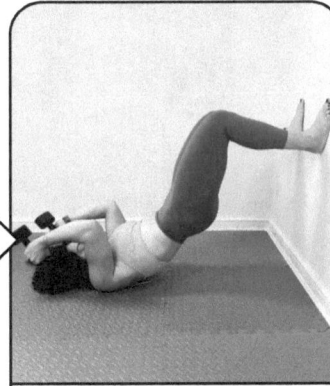

FINISH

🕐 **30 sec**

MUSCLE TONING - ARMS 2

DURATION:

4 min

GOAL:

Muscle Toning
and Endurance

1. HUG THE TREE
(PAGE 80)

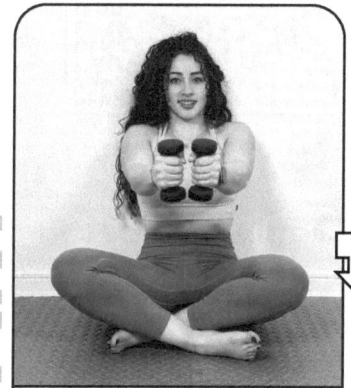

START

🕐 **30 sec**

2. WALL NARROW PUSH-UPS (PAGE 72)

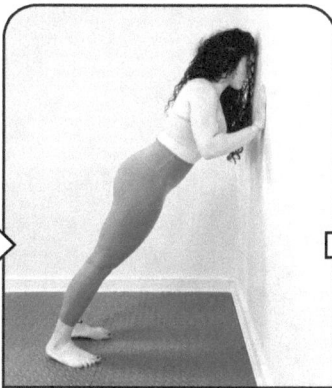

🕐 **30 sec**

3. SERVE A PLATTER
(PAGE 82)

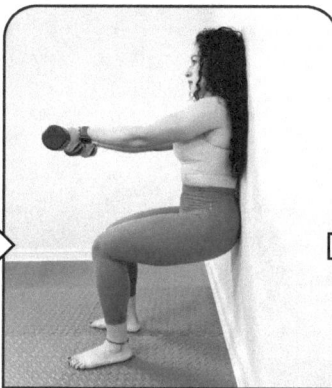

🕐 **30 sec**

4. REST

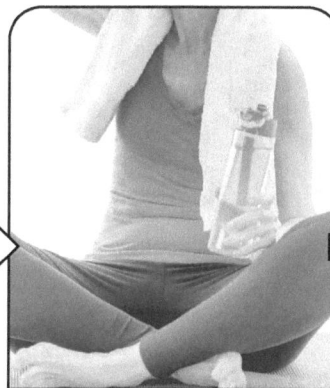

🕐 **30 sec**

5. WALL PUSH-UPS
(PAGE 70)

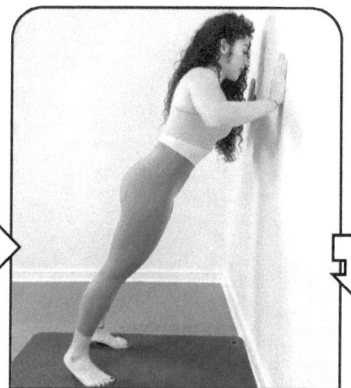

🕐 **30 sec**

6. SHOULDER PRESS + ALT HEELS (PAGE 76)

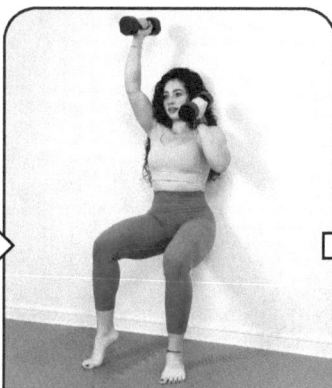

🕐 **30 sec**

7. CHEST PRESS BRIDGE (PAGE 78)

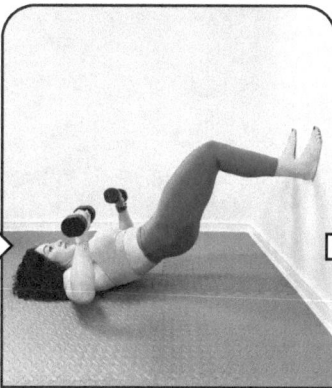

🕐 **30 sec**

8. SKULL CRUSHERS
(PAGE 84)

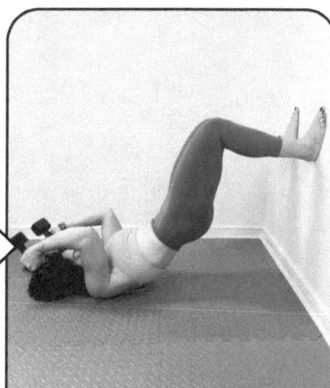

FINISH

🕐 **30 sec**

MUSCLE TONING - CORE 1

⏱ DURATION:
5 min 30 sec

◎ GOAL:
Muscle Toning and Endurance

START

1. AB CRUNCH + MARCH (PAGE 60)

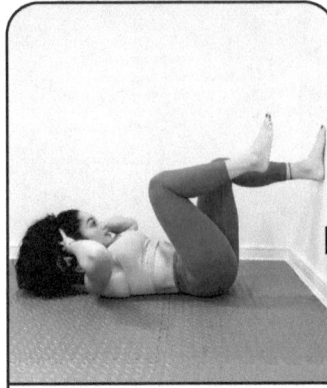

⏱ **30 sec**

2. THE HUNDREDS (PAGE 14)

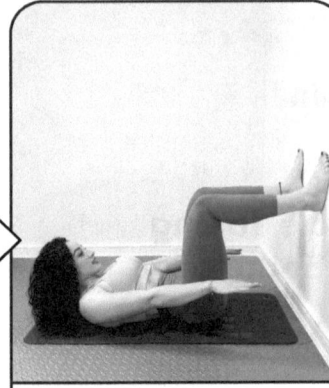

⏱ **30 sec**

3. FLEX UP ALTERNATE ARMS (PAGE 58)

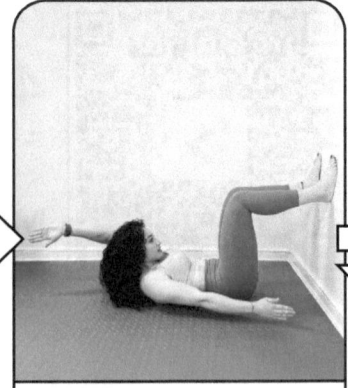

⏱ **30 sec**

4. REST

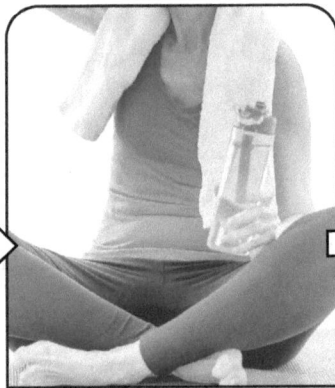

⏱ **30 sec**

5. MARCHING BRIDGE (PAGE 44)

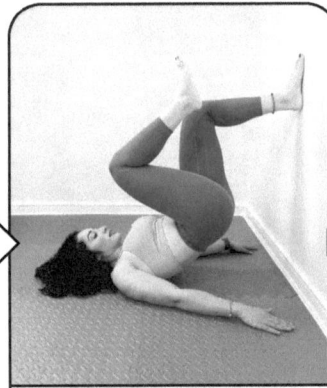

⏱ **30 sec**

6. TIPS UP TO HEEL (PAGE 62)

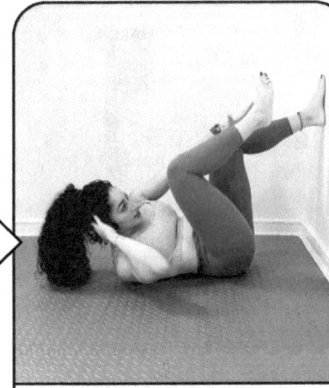

⏱ **30 sec**

7. TWIST TO KNEE (PAGE 56)

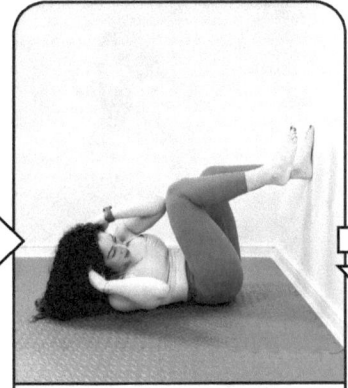

⏱ **30 sec**

8. REST

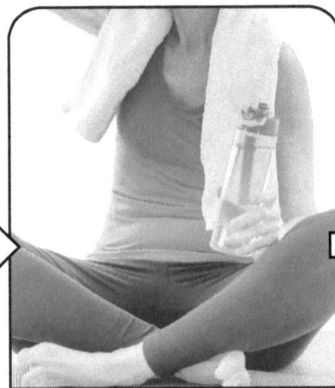

⏱ **30 sec**

9. SINGLE LEG LIFTS LEFT (PAGE 42)

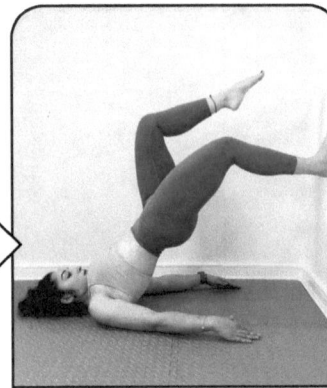

⏱ **30 sec**

10. SINGLE LEG LIFTS RIGHT (P. 42)

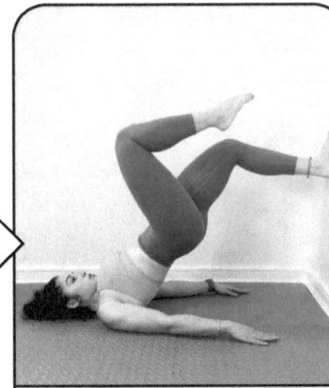

⏱ **30 sec**

11. BRIDGE AND KICK (PAGE 46)

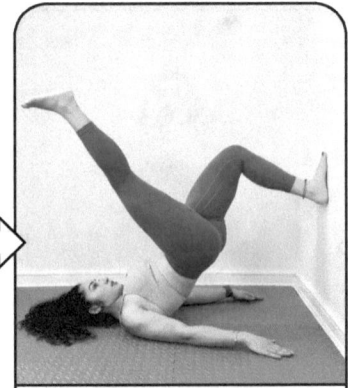

⏱ **30 sec**

FINISH

MUSCLE TONING - CORE 2

⟳ **DURATION:**

5 min

◎ **GOAL:**

Muscle Toning, Endurance and Flexibility

1. FLEX UP TO TOES
(PAGE 54)

2. TWIST TO KNEE
(PAGE 56)

START

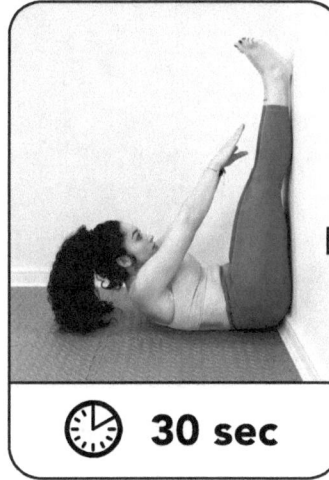

🕐 **30 sec**

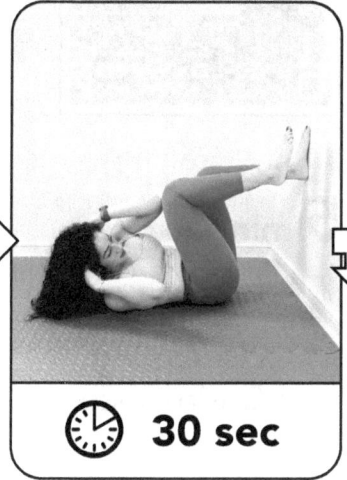

🕐 **30 sec**

3. REST

4. LEG CIRCLES LEFT
(PAGE 40)

5. LEG CIRCLES RIGHT
(PAGE 40)

**6. SINGLE LEG LIFTS
LEFT** (PAGE 42)

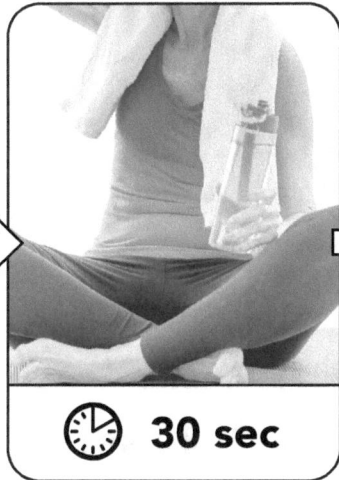

🕐 **30 sec**

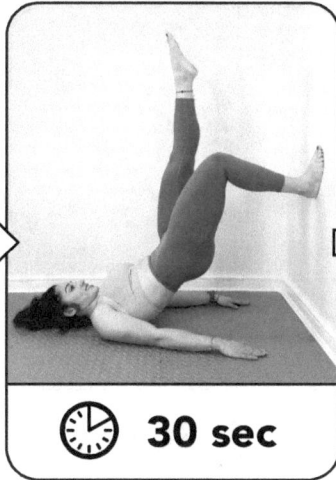

🕐 **30 sec**

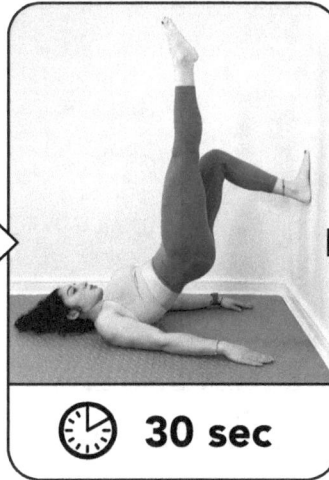

🕐 **30 sec**

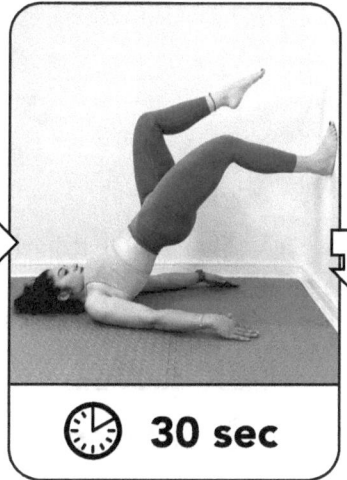

🕐 **30 sec**

**7. SINGLE LEG LIFTS
RIGHT** (PAGE 42)

8. REST

9. TIPS UP TO HEEL
(PAGE 62)

**10. MARCHING
BRIDGE** (PAGE 44)

FINISH

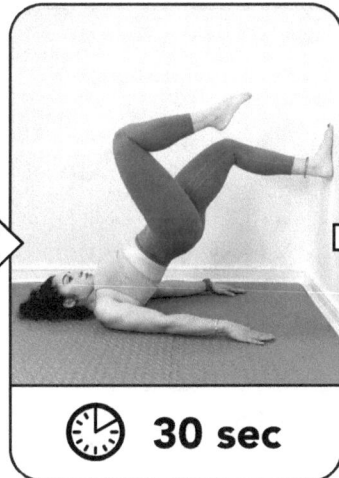

🕐 **30 sec**

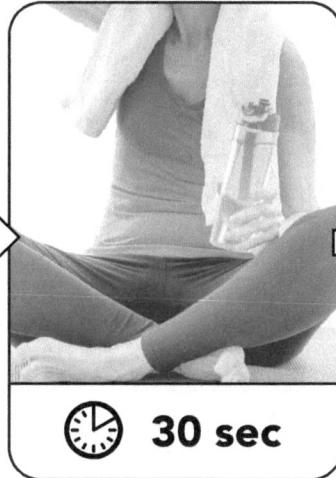

🕐 **30 sec**

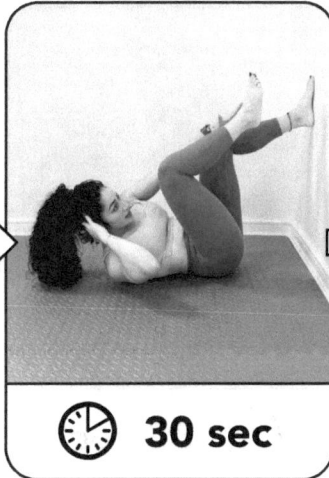

🕐 **30 sec**

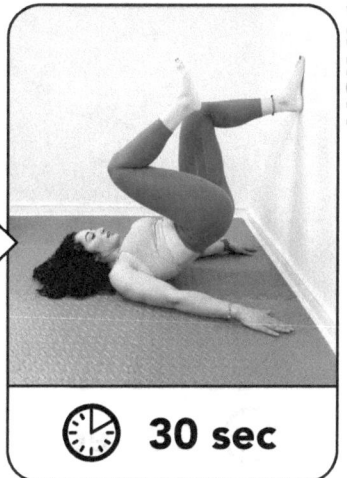

🕐 **30 sec**

MUSCLE TONING - CORE 3

START

1. HIP LIFTS
(PAGE 38)

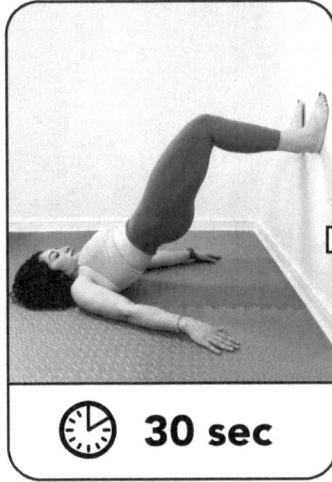

⏰ **30 sec**

2. MARCHING BRIDGE
(PAGE 44)

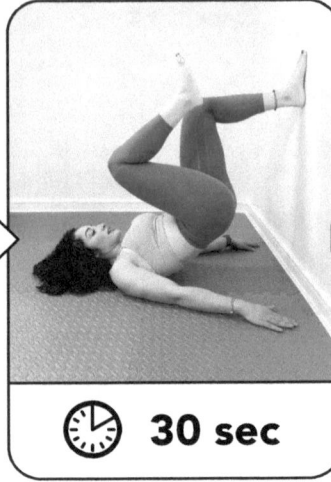

⏰ **30 sec**

3. REST

⏰ **30 sec**

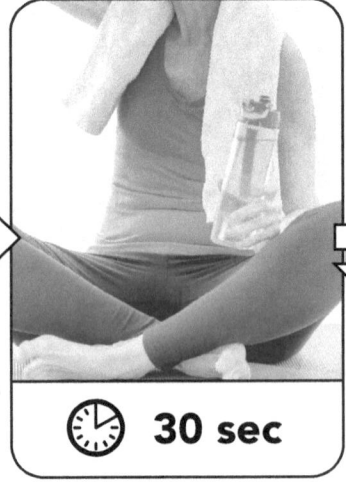

4. TWIST TO KNEE
(PAGE 56)

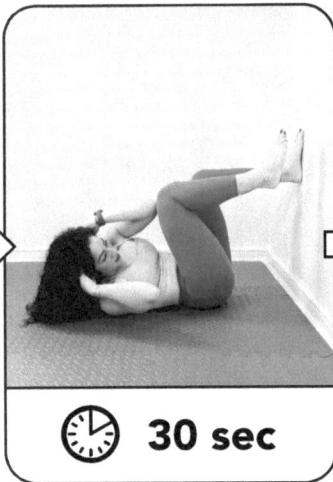

⏰ **30 sec**

5. MARCHING BRIDGE
(PAGE 44)

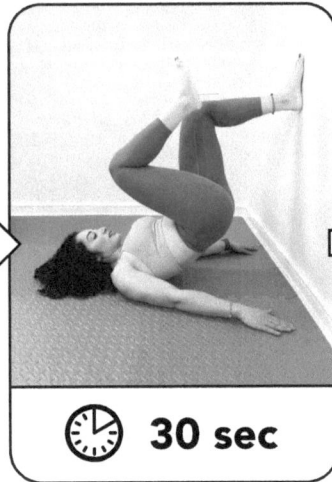

⏰ **30 sec**

6. REST

⏰ **30 sec**

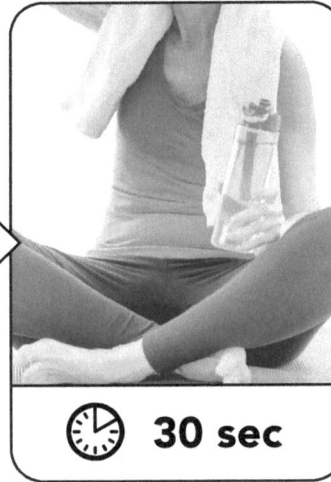

7. FLEX UP ALTERNATE ARMS (PAGE 58)

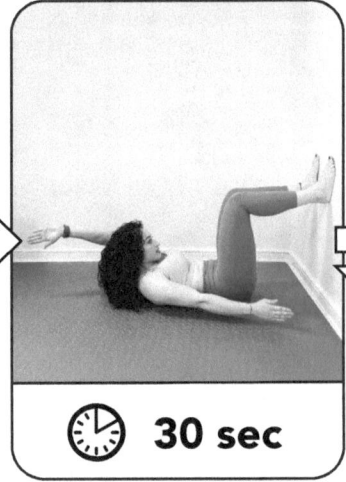

⏰ **30 sec**

8. MARCHING BRIDGE
(PAGE 44)

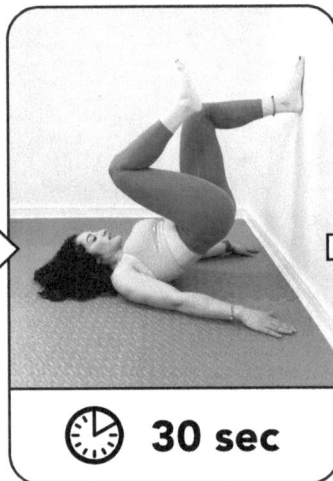

⏰ **30 sec**

9. REST

⏰ **30 sec**

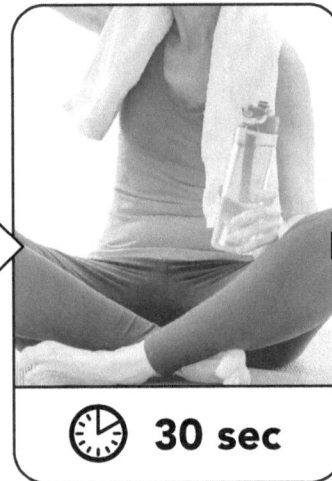

10. SINGLE LEG LIFTS LEFT (PAGE 42)

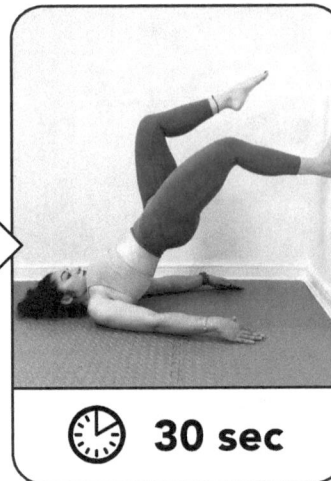

⏰ **30 sec**

11. SINGLE LEG LIFTS RIGHT (P. 42)

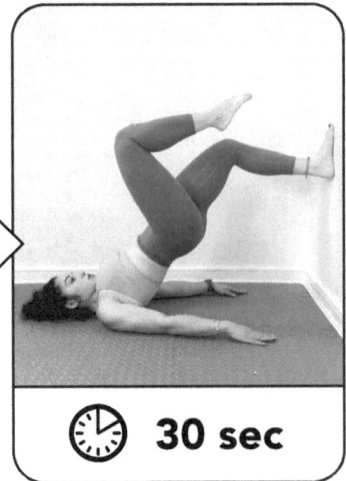

⏰ **30 sec**

FINISH

MUSCLE TONING - FULL BODY 1

⏱ DURATION:
4 min **30** sec

🎯 GOAL:
Muscle Toning and Endurance

1. SHOULDER PRESS + ALT HEELS (PAGE 76)

(PAGE 76)

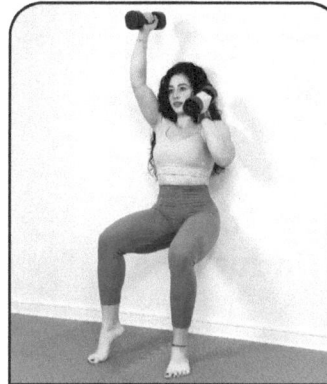

START

🕐 **30 sec**

2. WALL SIT HEEL RAISE (PAGE 13)

(PAGE 13)

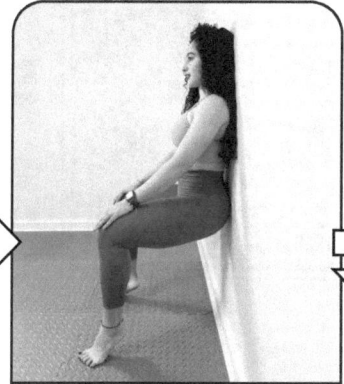

🕐 **30 sec**

3. WALL CHILD TO PLANK (PAGE 64)

(PAGE 64)

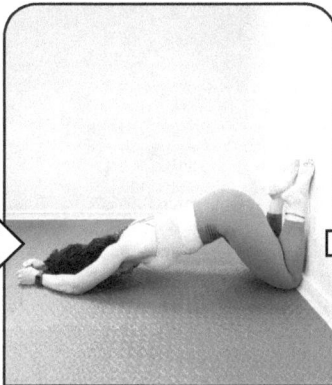

🕐 **30 sec**

4. REST

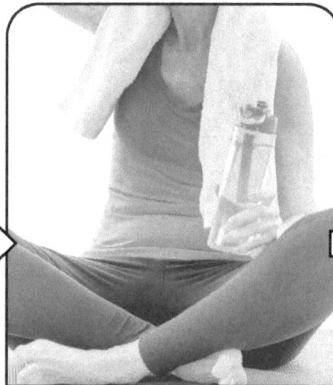

🕐 **30 sec**

5. HIP LIFTS (PAGE 38)

(PAGE 38)

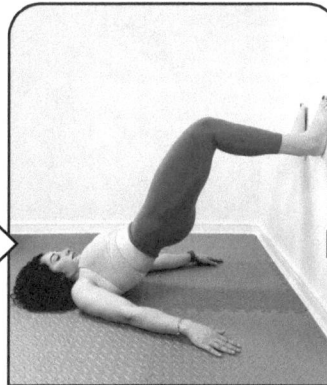

🕐 **30 sec**

6. SKULL CRUSHERS (PAGE 84)

(PAGE 84)

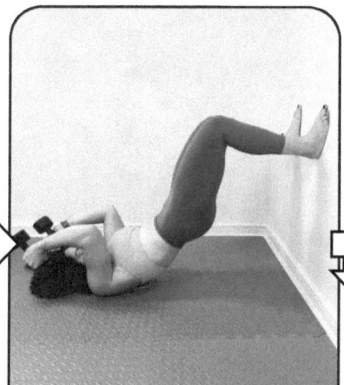

🕐 **30 sec**

7. SERVE A PLATTER (PAGE 82)

(PAGE 82)

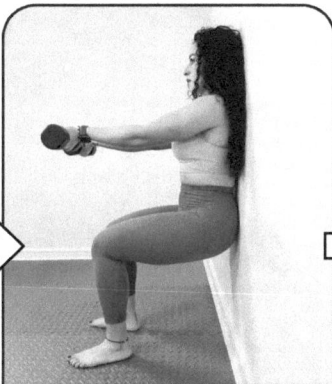

🕐 **30 sec**

8. TWIST TO KNEE (PAGE 56)

(PAGE 56)

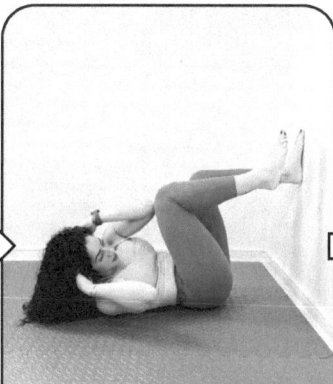

🕐 **30 sec**

9. MARCHING BRIDGE (PAGE 44)

(PAGE 44)

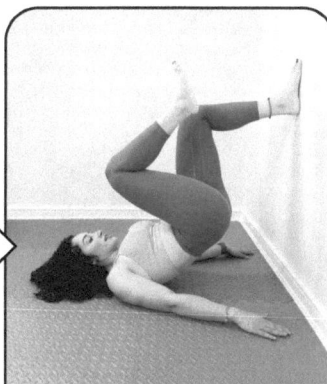

FINISH

🕐 **30 sec**

MUSCLE TONING - FULL BODY 2

⏱ **DURATION:**

5 min

🎯 **GOAL:**

Muscle Toning and Endurance

START

1. WALL SIT
(PAGE 12)

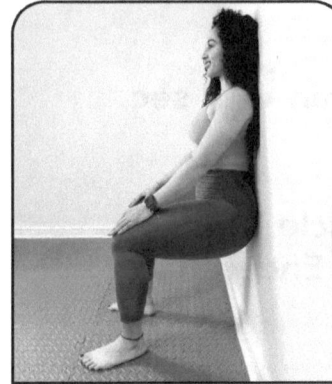

🕐 **HOLD 30 sec**

2. WALL-SUPPORTED KNEE RAISE (PAGE 66)

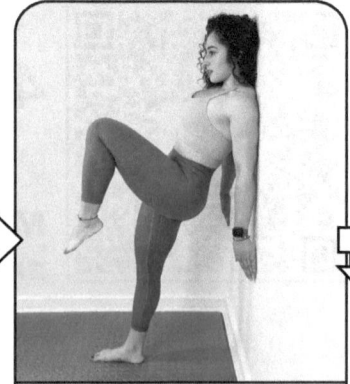

🕐 **30 sec**

3. WALL SIT HEEL RAISE (PAGE 13)

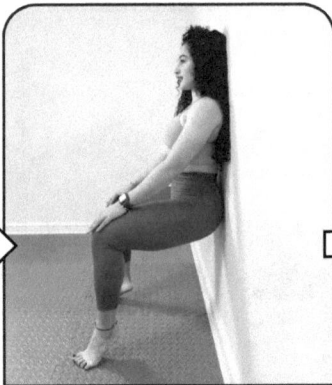

🕐 **30 sec**

4. WALL PUSH-UPS
(PAGE 70)

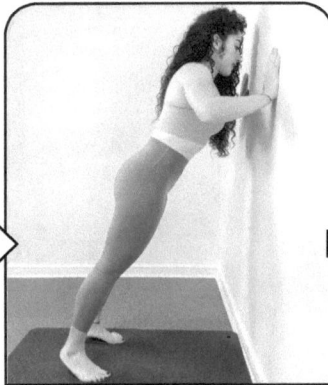

🕐 **30 sec**

5. WALL PLANK UPS
(PAGE 50)

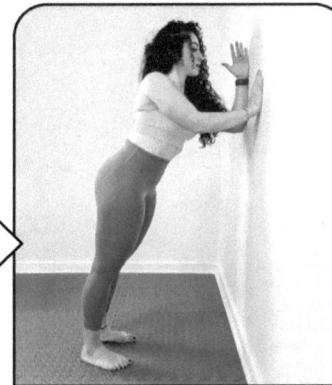

🕐 **30 sec**

6. TIPS UP TO HEEL
(PAGE 62)

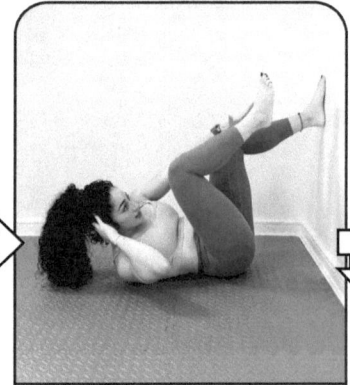

🕐 **30 sec**

7. REST

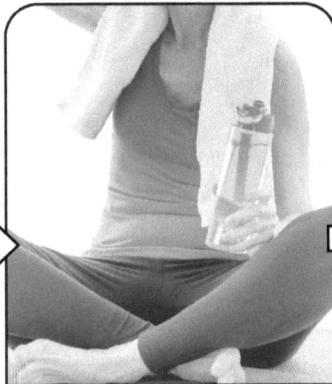

🕐 **30 sec**

8. AB CRUNCH + MARCH (PAGE 60)

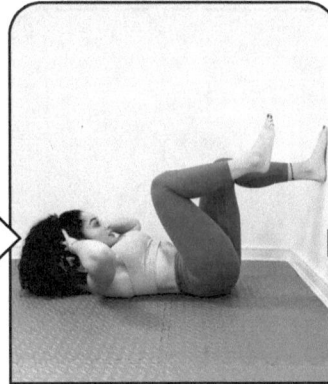

🕐 **30 sec**

9. THE HUNDREDS
(PAGE 14)

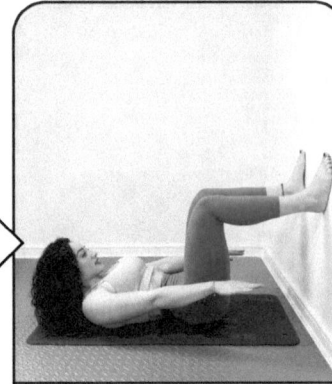

🕐 **30 sec**

10. MARCHING BRIDGE (PAGE 44)

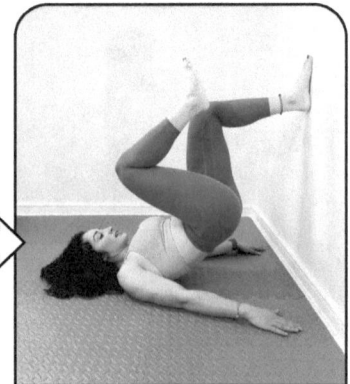

🕐 **30 sec**

FINISH

MUSCLE TONING - FULL BODY 3

⏱ **DURATION:**
5 min 30 sec

🎯 **GOAL:**
Muscle Toning and Endurance

START

1. WALL PUSH-UPS
(PAGE 70)

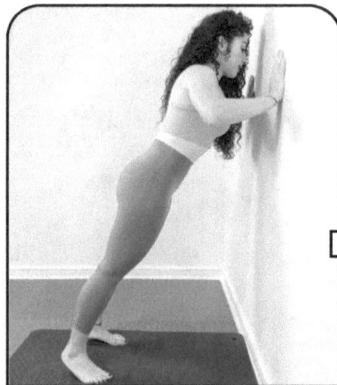

🕐 **30 sec**

2. WALL PLANK UPS
(PAGE 50)

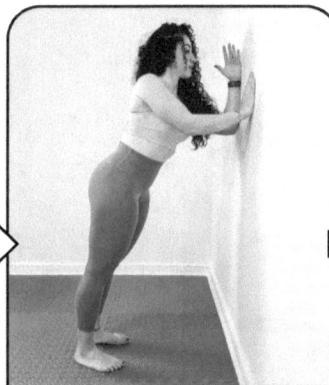

🕐 **30 sec**

3. SHOULDER PRESS + ALT HEELS (PAGE 76)

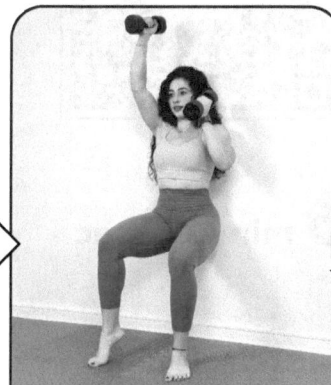

🕐 **30 sec**

4. REST

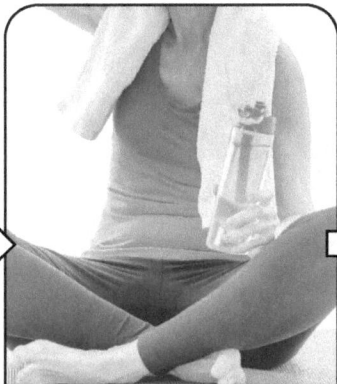

🕐 **30 sec**

5. HIP LIFTS
(PAGE 38)

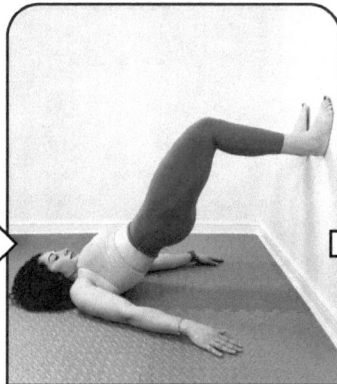

🕐 **30 sec**

6. SKULL CRUSHERS
(PAGE 84)

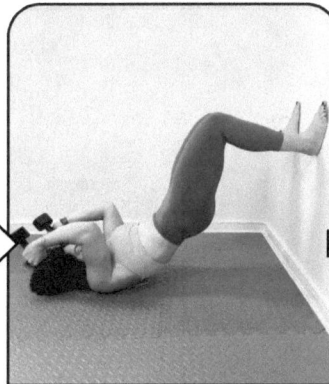

🕐 **30 sec**

7. TIPS UP TO HEEL
(PAGE 62)

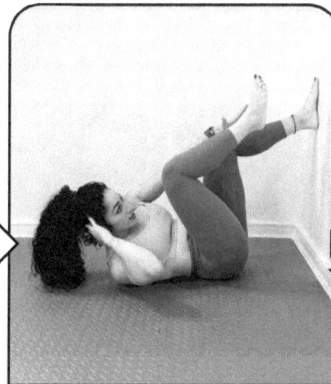

🕐 **30 sec**

8. REST

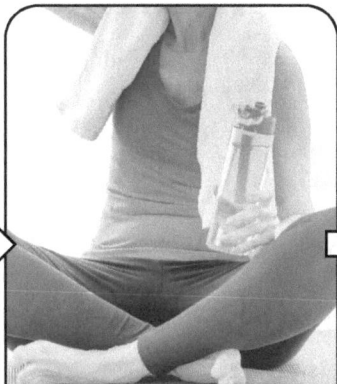

🕐 **30 sec**

9. WALL SIT
(PAGE 12)

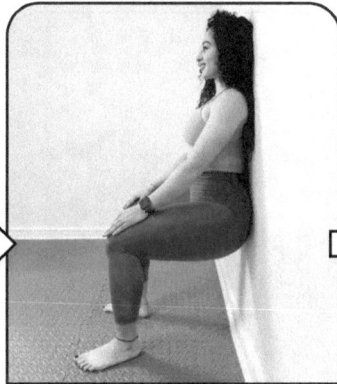

🕐 **HOLD 30 sec**

10. MARCHING BRIDGE (PAGE 44)

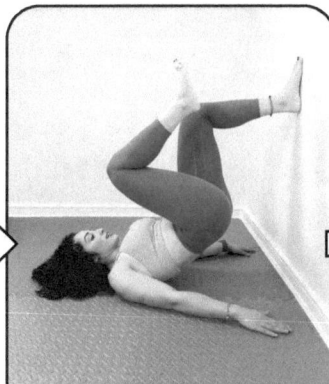

🕐 **30 sec**

11. THE HUNDREDS
(PAGE 14)

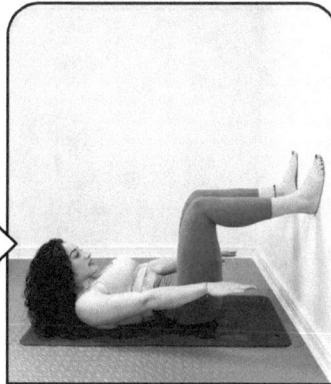

🕐 **30 sec**

FINISH

MUSCLE TONING - FULL BODY 4

DURATION:
5 min 30 sec

GOAL:
Muscle Toning

START

1. SIT & TWIST
(PAGE 86)

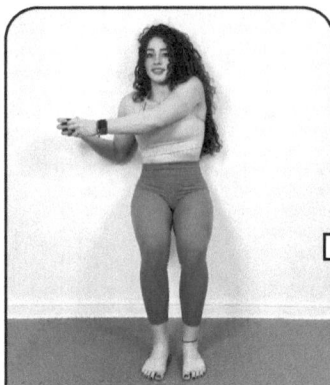

🕐 **30 sec**

2. W.S. DONKEY KICK LEFT (PAGE 68)

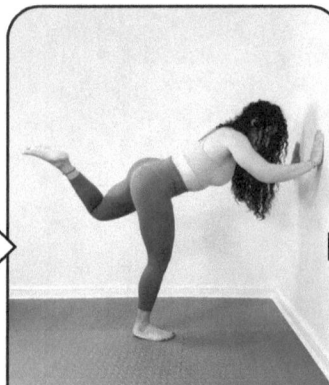

🕐 **30 sec**

3. W.S. DONKEY KICK RIGHT (PAGE 68)

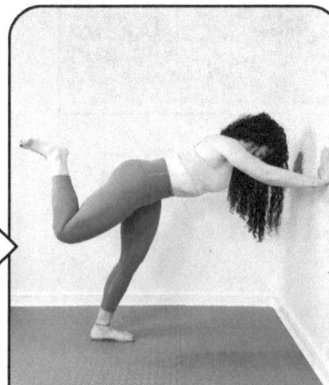

🕐 **30 sec**

4. MARCHING BRIDGE
(PAGE 44)

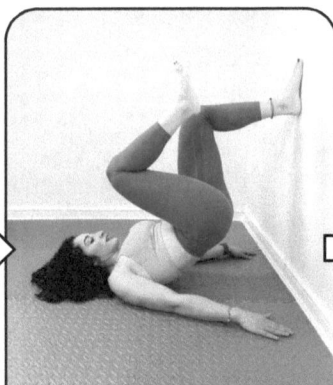

🕐 **30 sec**

5. BRIDGE AND KICK
(PAGE 46)

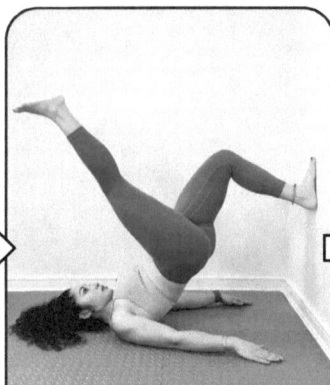

🕐 **30 sec**

6. REST

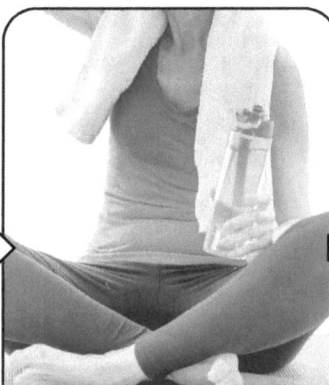

🕐 **30 sec**

7. WALL CHILD TO PLANK (PAGE 64)

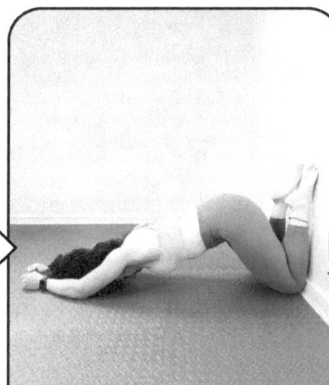

🕐 **30 sec**

8. FLEX UP TO TOES
(PAGE 54)

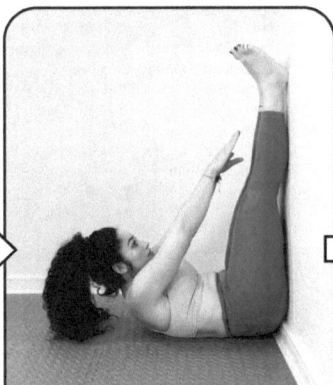

🕐 **30 sec**

9. CHEST PRESS BRIDGE (PAGE 78)

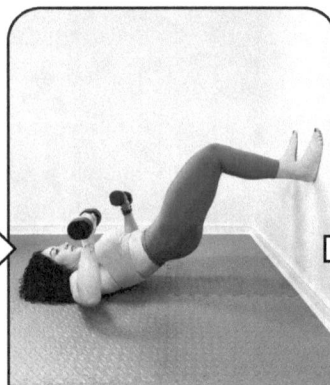

🕐 **30 sec**

10. SKULL CRUSHERS
(PAGE 84)

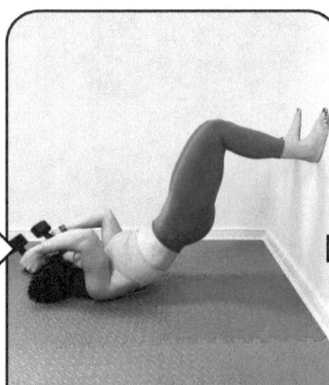

🕐 **30 sec**

11. SHOULDER PRESS + ALT HEELS (PAGE 76)

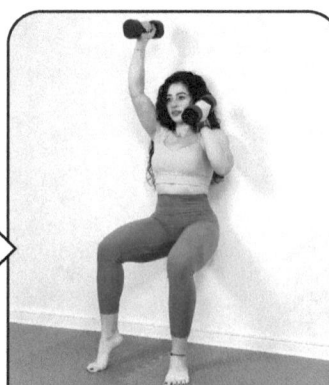

🕐 **30 sec**

FINISH

MUSCLE TONING - FULL BODY 5

⏱ DURATION:
5 min 30 sec

🎯 GOAL:
Muscle Toning and Endurance

START

1. SHOULDER PRESS + ALT HEELS (PAGE 76)

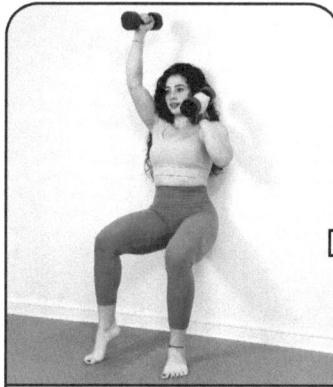

🕐 **30 sec**

2. WALL PUSH-UPS (PAGE 70)

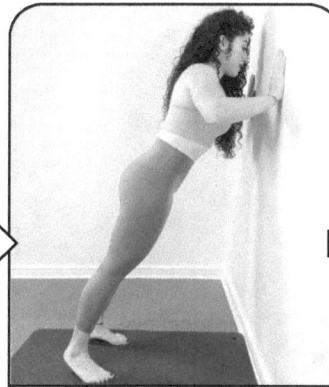

🕐 **30 sec**

3. REST

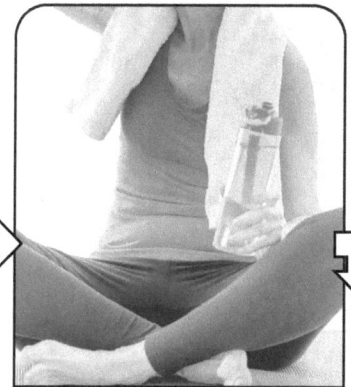

🕐 **30 sec**

4. WALL SIT (PAGE 12)

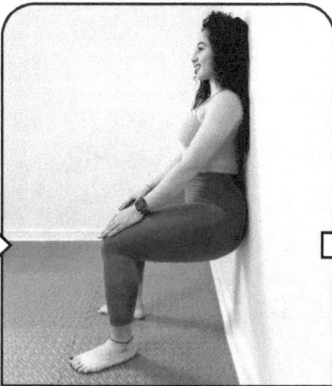

🕐 **HOLD 30 sec**

5. WALL PLANK UPS (PAGE 50)

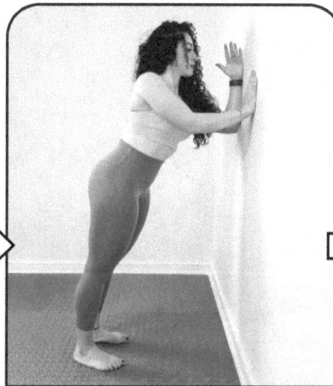

🕐 **30 sec**

6. REST

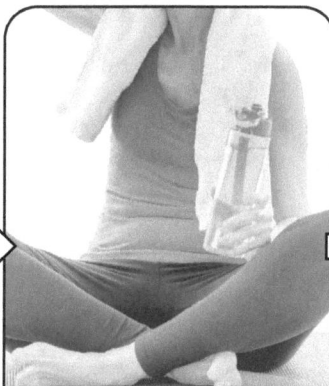

🕐 **30 sec**

7. WALL SIT KICKS (PAGE 48)

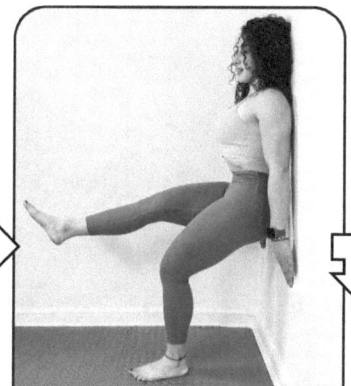

🕐 **30 sec**

8. SHOULDER TAPS (PAGE 52)

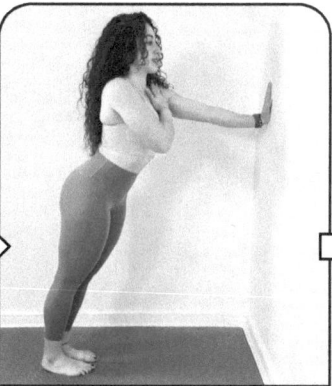

🕐 **30 sec**

9. REST

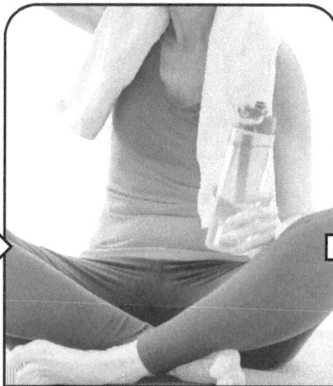

🕐 **30 sec**

10. MARCHING BRIDGE (PAGE 44)

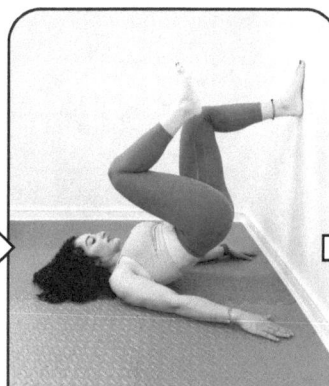

🕐 **30 sec**

11. BRIDGE AND KICK (PAGE 46)

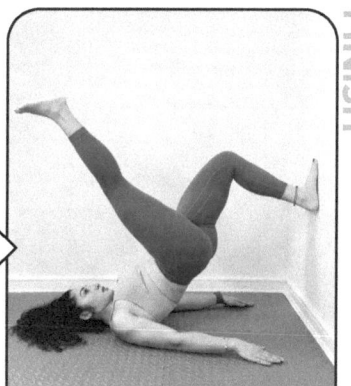

🕐 **30 sec**

FINISH

MUSCLE TONING - FULL BODY 6

DURATION:
5 min 30 sec

GOAL:
Muscle Toning and Endurance

START

1. SIT & TWIST
(PAGE 86)

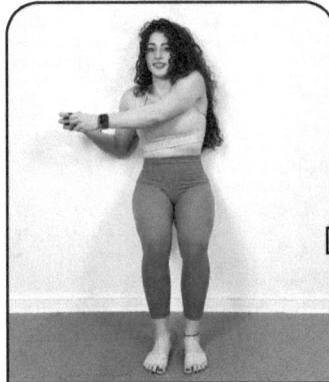

🕐 **30 sec**

2. WALL NARROW PUSH-UPS (PAGE 72)

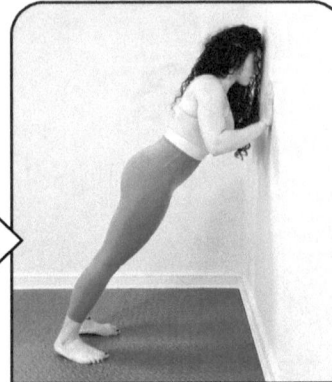

🕐 **30 sec**

3. LEG CIRCLES LEFT
(PAGE 40)

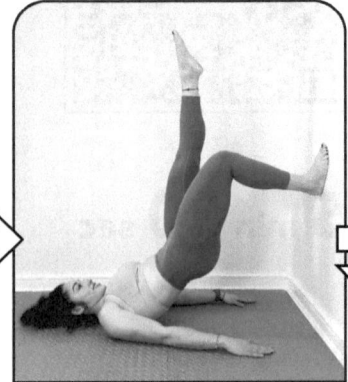

🕐 **30 sec**

4. LEG CIRCLES RIGHT
(PAGE 40)

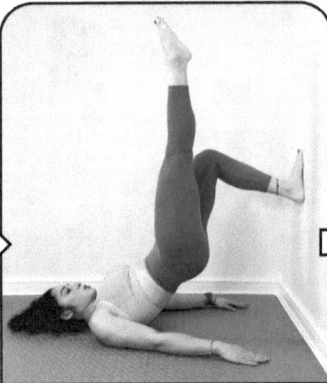

🕐 **30 sec**

5. REST

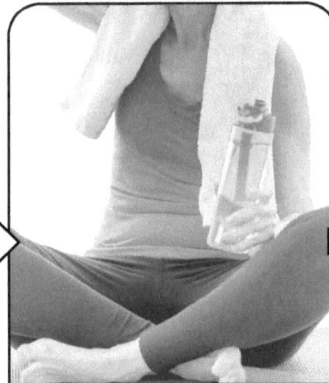

🕐 **30 sec**

6. SINGLE LEG LIFTS LEFT (PAGE 42)

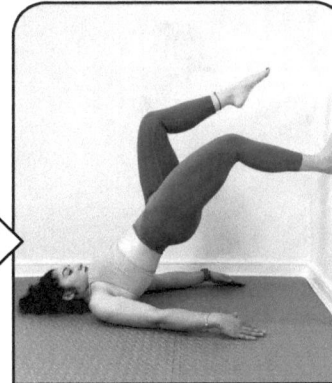

🕐 **30 sec**

7. SINGLE LEG LIFTS RIGHT (P. 42)

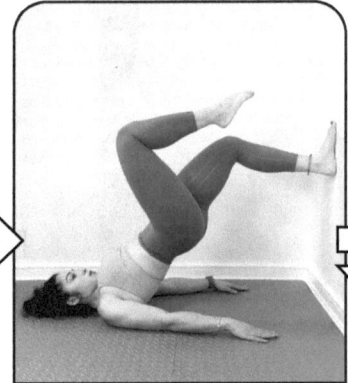

🕐 **30 sec**

8. WALL CHILD TO PLANK (PAGE 64)

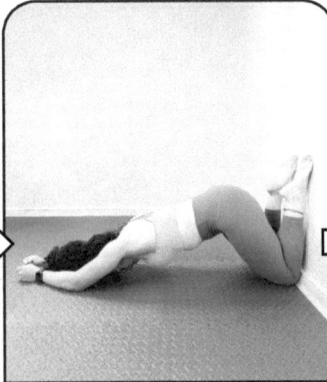

🕐 **30 sec**

9. FLEX UP TO TOES
(PAGE 54)

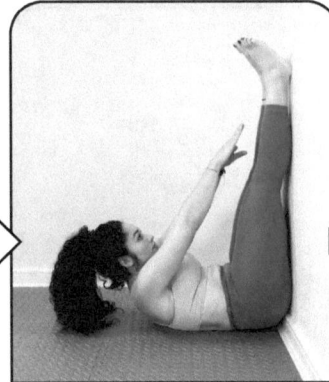

🕐 **30 sec**

10. WALL PUSH-UPS
(PAGE 70)

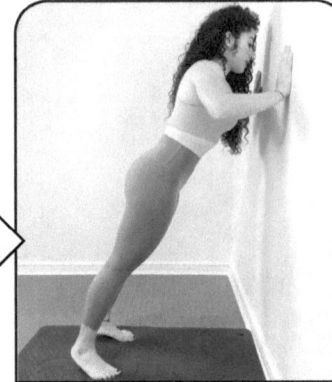

🕐 **30 sec**

11. WALL SIT
(PAGE 12)

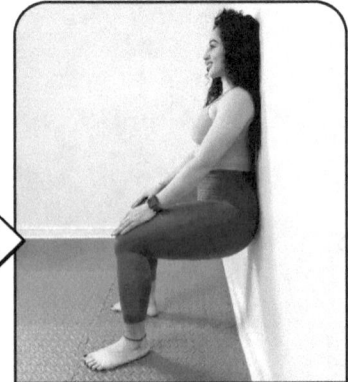

🕐 **HOLD 30 sec**

FINISH

28-DAY CHALLENGE

HOW TO APPROACH THE 28-DAY CHALLENGE

By taking on the 28-day Wall Pilates challenge, you're making a significant investment in your health and wellness. As you embark on this transformative path, remember these crucial elements to maximize the benefits of your journey:

Perseverance is Key: The core of this challenge is consistent engagement. To unlock the real benefits of Wall Pilates, make it a non-negotiable part of your daily routine. Select a time that suits you best, morning or night, and stick with it. This commitment not only builds discipline but also yields continuous improvements across various aspects of your fitness.

Body Awareness: While maintaining a routine is vital, it's equally essential to heed your body's cues. You may find yourself brimming with energy and eager for challenging moves on some days, yet on others, a gentler routine may suit you better. It is crucial to remember that the goal isn't to push yourself relentlessly but to honor and respond to your body's needs.

Prioritize Your Goals: Whether your aim is weight loss or enhancing your fitness, remember your purpose. On days when your drive diminishes, recall the commitment you made and the reasons behind undertaking this challenge. Envision your success—a healthier, more agile you—which can reignite your motivation and propel you forward on challenging days.

Envision Success: Picture the joy and pride you'll feel on day 28. Visualization is a potent motivational tool. Reflect on the gains in flexibility and strength you'll witness, and the gratification of reaching your goal. This mental image will inspire perseverance and add joy to your journey.

Embrace the Challenges: Throughout this journey, expect some days to be more demanding than others. These are crucial moments that test your resolve and contribute to your growth. When adversity strikes, reinforce your commitment and recognize your progress. Overcoming these challenges is a testament to your determination, edging you closer to your objectives.

Remember, each workout brings you closer to the version of yourself you aspire to be. Keep up the great work, stay persistent, and you will attain your fitness objectives. Believe in your strength, relish the journey, and celebrate every victory, no matter how small. You've got this!

N.B.: This book's 28-day challenge provides a daily warm-up and workout routine. Feel free to repeat the workout 1 to 3 times, depending on your fitness level.

28-DAY CHALLENGE

DAY 1
WORKOUT*:
M.T. - Full Body 1 (P. 101)

COOL DOWN:
Stretching 2 (P. 90)

DAY 2
WORKOUT*:
M.T. - Legs 1 (P. 94)

COOL DOWN:
Stretching 3 (P. 91)

DAY 3
WORKOUT*:
M.T. - Arms 1 (P. 96)

COOL DOWN:
Stretching 2 (P. 90)

DAY 4
REST

OR

Posture
Improvement 1 (P. 92)

DAY 5
WORKOUT*:
M.T. - Full Body 2 (P. 102)

COOL DOWN:
Stretching 1 (P. 89)

DAY 6
WORKOUT*:
M.T. - Core 1 (P. 98)

COOL DOWN:
Stretching 3 (P. 91)

DAY 7
REST

DAY 8
WORKOUT*:
M.T. - Full Body 3 (P. 103)

COOL DOWN:
Stretching 2 (P. 90)

DAY 9
WORKOUT*:
M.T. - Legs 2 (P. 95)

COOL DOWN:
Stretching 3 (P. 91)

DAY 10
WORKOUT*:
M.T. - Arms 2 (P. 97)

COOL DOWN:
Stretching 2 (P. 90)

DAY 11
REST

OR

Posture
Improvement 2 (P. 93)

DAY 12
WORKOUT*:
M.T. - Full Body 4 (P. 104)

COOL DOWN:
Stretching 2 (P. 90)

DAY 13
WORKOUT*:
M.T. - Core 2 (P. 99)

COOL DOWN:
Stretching 1 (P. 89)

DAY 14
REST

*Repeat the daily workout from 1 to 3 times, depending on your fitness level.

DAY 15

WORKOUT*:
M.T. - Full Body 5 (P. 105)

COOL DOWN:
Stretching 2 (P. 90)

DAY 16

WORKOUT*:
M.T. - Legs 1 (P. 94)

COOL DOWN:
Stretching 3 (P. 91)

DAY 17

WORKOUT*:
M.T. - Arms 1 (P. 96)

COOL DOWN:
Stretching 2 (P. 90)

DAY 18

REST

OR

Posture Improvement 1 (P. 92)

DAY 19

WORKOUT*:
M.T. - Full Body 6 (P. 106)

COOL DOWN:
Stretching 1 (P. 89)

DAY 20

WORKOUT*:
M.T. - Core 3 (P. 100)

COOL DOWN:
Stretching 3 (P. 91)

DAY 21

REST

DAY 22

WORKOUT*:
M.T. - Full Body 4 (P. 104)

COOL DOWN:
Stretching 2 (P. 90)

DAY 23

WORKOUT*:
M.T. - Legs 2 (P. 95)

COOL DOWN:
Stretching 3 (P. 91)

DAY 24

WORKOUT*:
M.T. - Arms 2 (P. 97)

COOL DOWN:
Stretching 2 (P. 90)

DAY 25

REST

OR

Posture Improvement 2 (P. 93)

DAY 26

WORKOUT*:
M.T. - Full Body 1 (P. 101)

COOL DOWN:
Stretching 2 (P. 90)

DAY 27

WORKOUT*:
M.T. - Core 1 (P. 98)

COOL DOWN:
Stretching 1 (P. 89)

DAY 28

REST

YOUR ACCESS CODE

232425

Thank you for choosing "Wall Pilates Workouts For Women." We're excited to help you embark on your wall pilates journey!

To access our exclusive online platform, where you'll discover video tutorials for exercises, routines, and workouts designed to complement the content of this book, please follow these simple steps:

STEP 1: Visit our website **www.sheerfitnessvibes.com** and navigate to the 'wall-pilates' section. You can access this platform on your <u>computer, tablet, or smartphone</u>.

STEP 2: In this section, a pop-up should appear, asking for an 'Access Code.' Enter the code **232425** into the provided field, and the pop-up should disappear, allowing you to access the section.

STEP 3: Enjoy Your Content! Now that you have entered the code, you'll gain full access to all the wall pilates exercises, routines, and workouts corresponding to this book. Explore the platform and enjoy the benefits of wall pilates at your own pace.

> ⚠ **Important Notes:**
> If you use a different device or browser to access our website, you may need to re-enter the code.

Thank you for being a part of our fitness community. We're here to support you on your wellness journey, and we hope you find our platform a valuable resource to enhance your practice.

If you encounter any issues with your access code or need assistance, please don't hesitate to contact our support team at support@sheerfitnessvibes.com.

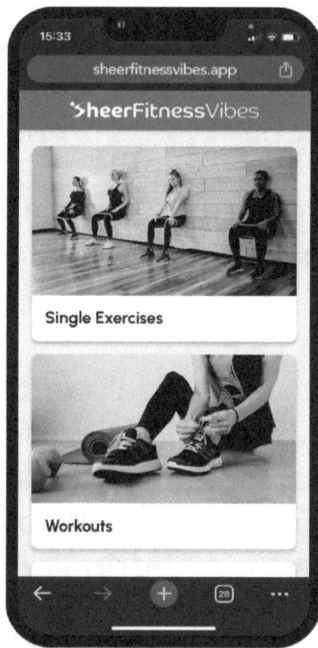

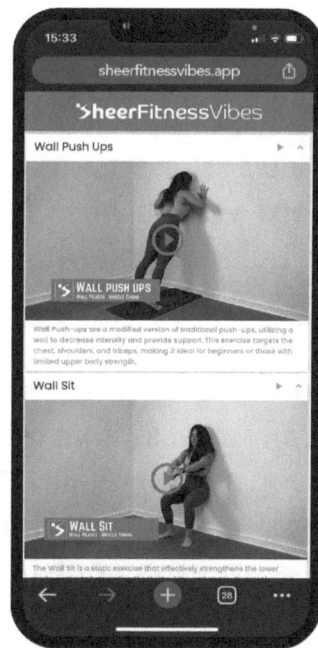

ENJOY OUR APP!

We are excited to introduce our Sheer Fitness Vibes app, designed specifically for phones and tablets. Keep your workouts always within reach on your device! Download it for Android or Apple by scanning the QR codes below.

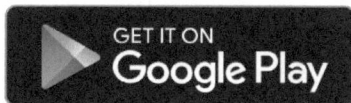

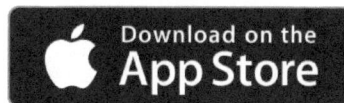

Not ready to download? You can still experience our app online. Save storage and preview the app via our web version. For more info, visit:
www.sheerfitnessvibes.com/appsetup

BONUS

As a special thank you for choosing our book, we're excited to present an exclusive bonus to complement your fitness routine. Introducing "Intermittent Fasting After 50" - a digital guide tailored to enhance your health and amplify the benefits of your wall pilates practice.

We firmly believe in the power of wall pilates as a standalone tool for weight loss and improving overall fitness. If you find fulfillment and progress through the practices alone, that's wonderful! Wall Pilates is a complete and effective approach in itself. However, if you're curious about amplifying your results and exploring other safe health strategies, intermittent fasting might be an intriguing addition.

Intermittent fasting isn't just a diet trend; it's a sustainable lifestyle change that has been shown to offer numerous health benefits, including improved metabolic health, increased cognitive function, and enhanced physical energy. When combined with the gentle yet effective exercises in wall pilates, intermittent fasting can be a powerful tool in managing your weight and improving overall health.

This guide provides actionable strategies and tips to safely integrate intermittent fasting into your lifestyle. Whether you're a beginner to fasting or looking to refine your approach, "Intermittent Fasting After 50" is designed to be accessible and informative for all.

To access your free digital copy of "Intermittent Fasting After 50", simply scan the QR code below or visit the URL **https://bit.ly/4aN065S**. This exclusive content is our gift to you! It's a tool to empower and guide you as you continue your wellness journey with wall pilates.

https://bit.ly/4aN065S

Made in United States
Troutdale, OR
01/31/2025